A Manual of
FRACTURES
and
DISLOCATIONS

By BARBARA BARTLETT STIMSON
A.B., M.D., MED. SC.D., F.A.C.S.

Director of Department of Bone and Joint Surgery, St. Francis Hospital, Poughkeepsie, New York; Chairman of Trauma Committee, Vassar Brothers Hospital, Poughkeepsie, New York; Consultant in Orthopedics, Hudson River State Hospital, Poughkeepsie, New York; Sharon Hospital, Sharon, Connecticut; Northern Dutchess Health Center, Rhinebeck, New York; Formerly Assistant Professor of Surgery, Columbia Presbyterian Medical Center, and Attending Surgeon on the Fracture Service at Presbyterian Hospital

Third Edition, Thoroughly Revised

97 Illustrations

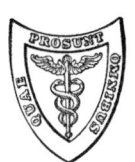

Lea & Febiger
PHILADELPHIA
1956

© by Lea & Febiger, 1956

Library of Congress Card Catalog Number 56-6931
Printed in The United States of America

Preface to the Third Edition

EIGHT years' experience in a small city away from a large teaching center has modified the author's viewpoint in several respects. As this small book is intended for students, internes, and general practitioners, it has been revised, it is hoped, with a better understanding of their needs and problems. No attempt has been made to describe operative techniques nor the detailed care of serious injuries. Such cases will, of necessity, be in the hands of specialists for definitive treatment. More emphasis has therefore been placed on the common injuries which are largely handled by the general practitioner. This book is in no way meant to replace the numerous volumes which treat the subject in detail, but if it provides some help in time of need, its existence will be justified.

B. B. S.

POUGHKEEPSIE, NEW YORK

Preface to the First Edition

THIS handbook is intended primarily for medical students, but it is hoped that general practitioners will find it of value. It is designed as a guide to the wealth of material that is published in textbooks and articles which bewilder the student with their mass of detail. No attempt has been made to make the book an exhaustive treatise; the student is referred to the standard texts for elaboration. Although fracture surgery is becoming a specialty, nevertheless every doctor, be he psychiatrist or obstetrician, will sooner or later encounter a fracture, possibly in his own household. The author hopes that this volume will give him the fundamental knowledge he may need without burdening him with the detailed information demanded of the expert.

Grateful acknowledgement is made of the unlimited time and assistance given by the members of the Staff of the Fracture Service of the Presbyterian Hospital, New York City. The author wishes particularly to express her gratitude to the illustrators, Anna K. Stimson and Martha G. Hunter, who, with tireless patience and skill, have labored to express in black and white her nebulous ideas. Without the painstaking secretarial aid of Jessie A. Harding this book might not have been written.

B. B. S.

NEW YORK CITY

Foreword

THAT a third edition of this book is necessary is unequivocal evidence that since 1939 earlier editions fulfilled their stated purpose; *viz.*, an instrument for the instruction of the student and a guide for the general practitioner. In the light of great advances in the surgery of trauma, the paucity of additions and changes required testifies to the basic rationale of its contents. The pattern remains as originally conceived, a simple text predicated upon the fundamentals of injury and repair. Both Dr. Stimson and this volume remain a cornerstone of the teaching program of the Fracture Service of The Presbyterian Hospital in New York City, and the third edition is heartily commended to all other teaching services.

Harrison L. McLaughlin, M.D., C.M.

Contents

CHAPTER   PAGE

PART I

General Considerations

1. Definition, Classification and Diagnosis of Fractures 9
2. Bone Repair in Fractures 19
3. Symptoms and Signs of Fractures 24
4. Principles of Treatment of Fractures . . . 29
5. Details of Technique in Treatment of Fractures 42
6. Accident Ward Procedure 58

PART II

The Upper Extremity

7. Injuries to the Shoulder Girdle 61
8. Injuries at the Shoulder Joint 74
9. Fractures of the Shaft of the Humerus . . . 91
10. Injuries at the Elbow Joint 94
11. Injuries to the Forearm 120
12. Injuries at the Wrist 124
13. Injuries to the Hand 138

PART III

The Trunk

14. Injuries to the Chest 147
15. Injuries to the Spine 148
16. Injuries to the Pelvic Girdle 154

PART IV

THE LOWER EXTREMITY

CHAPTER		PAGE
17.	Injuries at the Hip Joint	157
18.	Fractures of the Shaft of the Femur	173
19.	Injuries at the Knee Joint	178
20.	Fractures of the Shafts of the Tibia and Fibula	189
21.	Injuries at the Ankle Joint	194
22.	Injuries to the Foot	203

FRACTURES AND DISLOCATIONS

Part I. General Considerations

Chapter 1

Definition, Classification and Diagnosis of Fractures

DEFINITION OF FRACTURES

In spite of the amazing advances in preventive and therapeutic medicine that have been made during recent years, science has failed to prevent small boys from falling out of trees, elderly ladies from slipping on scatter rugs, or high-powered cars from crashing. Accidents resulting in fractures or dislocations occur in the home, in the playground, on the farm, in the factory, and on the highway with such frequency that it is essential that all doctors, regardless of specialty, should have a knowledge of the fundamental principles of treatment. In order to have such knowledge it is necessary to understand what is involved.

A fracture in its simplest terms is a broken bone: in scientific terminology "a solution of continuity of osseous tissue." A dislocation is the displacement of a bone at a joint or articulation.

But these definitions are not enough. A broken bone cannot be removed from its surroundings, fastened together with nails or glue and hung on the wall to dry. It must be treated as part of a living organism. It is an injury to an individual involving a certain portion of the body and must

10   Classification and Diagnosis of Fractures

be evaluated not as a separate entity but as part of a human being.

A fracture is an injury. It is not a disease with a slow onset nor is it a surgical operation of choice allowing preparation of mind and affairs. It is an emergency that usually occurs to individuals who in the midst of health are pursuing their occupations or pleasures. It comes without warning and, therefore, is associated with some degree of mental shock. Because it is an injury it is accompanied by trauma to other structures. A broken bone is not an isolated phenomenon; there are torn vessels, bruised muscles, lacerated periosteum, contused nerves; sometimes there are injured internal organs, sometimes lacerated skin. This soft part damage is always present to some extent and must be taken into consideration.

A fracture occurs in an individual. Frequently overlooked, this fact is of the utmost importance, for age, sex, and mode of living all influence the treatment and outcome of the case. Child, adult, or octogenarian, each presents his own problems. A slight deformity resulting from a broken clavicle may be unsightly with an evening dress but of no importance under a man's shirt. The patient's occupation must be considered. Is he a laborer or a pianist, a clerk or a watchmaker? Will he lose his job if he comes into the hospital for a few days or can he cut coupons just as well in a private room as he can in the office? The temperament of the patient must be recognized for it is necessary to know if he will carry out instructions intelligently, if he can be jollied, or if he must be bullied into obeying orders. So much of the functional result in fractures depends on the patient that his coöperation must be gained from the outset. In surgical cases, a cholecystectomy for example, with adequate surgical and nursing care the intestinal tract functions regardless of the patient. But in a fracture case the usefulness of the ex-

Classification and Diagnosis of Fractures 11

tremity depends on the patient himself, no matter how satisfactory the late x-ray pictures may be.

Two cases may serve to illustrate the foregoing. Two women slipped and fell on an icy sidewalk landing on their outstretched right hands. Both sustained fractures of the lower end of the right radius, Colles' fractures. Both went to the same doctor and the examination and x-ray pictures of each were strikingly similar. They received the same treatment of immediate reduction and immobilization with splints for the same period of time. One woman was the wife of a laborer with five children to look after and all the help she had was that which the neighbors gave her. From the first day she was moving her fingers and trying to help herself. She was sensible, rather stoical, and, having complete confidence in her doctor, she obeyed instructions when the splints were removed and used her hand and wrist. She had an excellent functional as well as anatomical result in a minimal space of time. The other woman was a society matron whose heaviest occupation was holding cards at bridge. She had a personal maid and refused to help herself in any way. When the splints were removed the fingers were swollen, stiff, and painful on attempted motion. Having heard that one of her friends had "electric treatments" for a similar injury, she demanded them, but as she expected the treatments to do all the work, she could not understand why her wrist and hand remained sore and stiff for weeks. The anatomical result was as good in the second case as it was in the first. The fractures were the same but the individuals were different.

A fracture involves a portion of the body. Different parts of the body have dissimilar functions and must be treated accordingly. The upper extremity has a wide range of motion and is capable of performing skilled and fine acts; mobility therefore must be preserved. The function of the lower extremity is static and progressive

12   Classification and Diagnosis of Fractures

weight-bearing, *i.e.*, standing and walking; axis, length and stability are essential. In a fracture of a phalanx of the finger every effort is directed toward retaining the motion of the finger if possible. A stiff finger-joint may be a serious economic handicap. A broken phalanx of a toe, on the contrary, is treated in such a way as to prevent a deformity

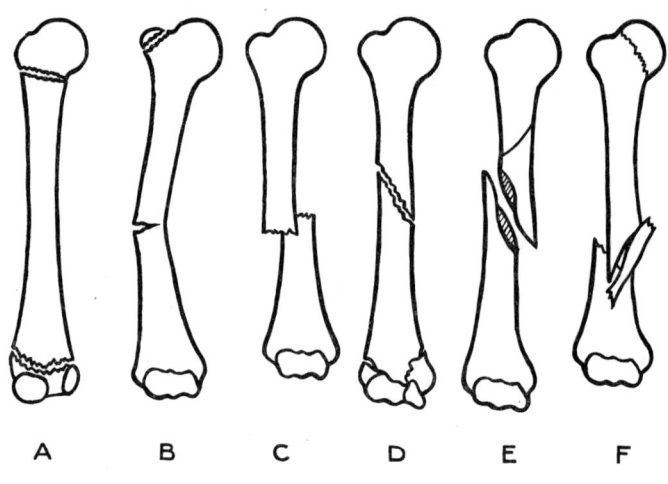

Fig. 1.—Types of fractures.

which might give pain on weight-bearing; limited motion in a toe joint is of relatively little importance.

Finally, a fracture is a break in a bone. The kind of bone involved, the location of the injury in the bone, and the character of the break are factors which must be taken into consideration in an intelligent choice of treatment.

CLASSIFICATION OF FRACTURES

Fractures are divided into two main groups, closed or simple, and open or compound. A fracture is called closed when there is no wound of the skin communicating with the break in the bone. A fracture is open when the break in

Classification and Diagnosis of Fractures

the bone communicates with the outside air through a wound in the skin and is therefore potentially infected.

A fracture may be a bend or a buckling in the bone; it may appear as a crack, a fissure, or a depression; it may be complete with the broken bone ends transverse, oblique, or spiral. It may consist of a small chip avulsed from the main bone or it may be comminuted, *i.e.*, consist of three or more fragments (Fig. 1).

Various kinds of displacements may occur. One fragment can be tilted on the other, causing an angulation in the contour of the bone. If the fracture is complete one fragment can shift on the other anteriorly, posteriorly, laterally or medially. It can also rotate. The lower fragment can be pushed upward or cephalad, becoming impacted if it is still in contact with the other fragment, or overriding it if it has moved the full width of the bone. It can be forced downward or caudad by massive swelling and hemorrhage or by overpull. Customarily the smaller fragment is said to be displaced on the larger or the distal on the proximal one.

DIAGNOSIS OF FRACTURES

The history of a fracture patient is usually so simple and straightforward that it is frequently very carelessly taken. "The man slipped and fell and hurt his arm," is unfortunately often seen on charts. Definite information must be obtained and certain questions asked. The time of the accident is important. Was it within an hour or was it a week ago? The place of the fall must be recorded and a special note made if the patient was working, because of the compensation laws. What was he doing at the time of injury? Walking, running, skating, etc.? How did he land? That is always a difficult question for a patient to answer, for a fall comes so unexpectedly that he finds himself suddenly on the ground and is rarely quite sure in what order he arrived there; too much credence should not be given to his story.

14   Classification and Diagnosis of Fractures

What happened next? This is of great interest and must be carefully investigated. Did he notice that his arm hurt at once or that he could not use it or that it looked crooked? If there was deformity it is important to know if a friend or bystander pulled on the arm and made it look better, *i.e.*, reduced a dislocation. Has he noticed any tingling, numbness, or lack of motion of his fingers, *i.e.*, is there a suggestion of nerve lesion? Has he tried any home remedies before coming to the doctor? It is valuable to know that the redness and blisters on the skin are due to overenthusiastic applications of iodine. Has he ever hurt that arm before? Frequently an old deformity will complicate the diagnosis of a fresh fracture if its existence is not suspected.

An elaborate and lengthy history is not necessary but all the salient facts, both negative and positive, must be written down both for the better treatment of the patient and for the sake of the doctor. Many of these cases are medicolegal and inadequate and inaccurate histories may prove embarrassing to the doctor on the witness stand or to subsequent doctors treating the case.

The examination of the patient must begin with a consideration of the individual. Is he in pain? Is he in shock? Sometimes only a cursory examination is possible before supportive measures are instituted in order to save life. This seems self-evident, but it is surprising how often the attention of students and internes is taken up with some obvious deformity to the neglect of the general condition of the patient. If he is not unconscious nor in shock it is important to make a quick estimate of the characteristics of the individual. Is he stoical or neurotic, frightened or in pain? The interpretation of the local examination must be based on this estimate to be of any real value.

The local examination must above all things be gentle. It need be no less painstaking and careful, but if the coöperation of the patient is lost at the beginning it may never be completely regained. This is particularly true with chil-

Classification and Diagnosis of Fractures 15

dren. It is wise to warn a child if you know some part of the examination will hurt. Never lie, for once a child's confidence is lost it is almost impossible to win back. Rough and thoughtless handling can also produce further damage to the soft tissue and to splintered bone ends.

Inspection will tell a great deal if the eyes are trained and know for what to look. Comparison of the two extremities should always be made, for failure to do so may cause a normal individual variation to be considered the result of a recent injury. *Deformity* or change in the contour due to change in the bony framework must be sought, and any deviation from the normal anatomical landmarks recognized and interpreted. Soft part *swelling* is frequently present and may mask slight deformity. *Ecchymosis* is the discoloration of skin caused by the underlying extravasation of blood and is suggestive of the existence of a fracture, especially if it is seen two or three days after the injury. It frequently appears at some distance from the site of the break in the bone because the blood from the bone ends passes down the fascial planes, gradually approaching the surface. Ecchymosis is seen sooner and nearer the fracture if there has been extensive tearing of the soft parts.

Palpation should begin well away from the obviously painful area. Occasionally the inexperienced doctor pounces on the sore spot with eager fingers, the patient naturally jerks away, and it is with considerable difficulty that the examination proceeds. Confidence must be gained by gentle handling and all painful procedures should be postponed as long as possible. Where no visible deformity has been seen, direct bony tenderness should be carefully mapped out. This can frequently be done by the patient himself if he is given a pencil and shown how to press the eraser end along the shaft of the bone until he finds the point or line that hurts the most. With care the line of the fracture can be traced on the skin. Indirect or transmitted tenderness is a sign of

16 Classification and Diagnosis of Fractures

importance to distinguish a break from a soft part lesion. It is elicited by gentle pressure on the extremities of a bone in the axis of its shaft. Bony irregularity can be felt even when masked by swelling. Bony crepitus and a false point of motion are definite evidences of the existence of a fracture but should never be elicited unless absolutely necessary to establish the diagnosis. To do so may cause extensive damage to soft parts and bone ends.

The condition of the circulation as manifested by the temperature and color of the extremity and the presence or absence of adjacent pulses should always be included in the initial examination. A rapid investigation of the sensory and motor functions will demonstrate the condition of the peripheral nerves and should not be omitted, for it is essential to know the extent of the damage as soon as possible. Vessels and nerves are occasionally injured during the course of treatment, and a note of the presence or absence of circulatory or neurological lesions existing before treatment is started may save both the patient and doctor from later difficulties.

The existence of other injuries must never be overlooked. It is possible to have two or more fractures in the same individual and it is embarrassing to find the second fracture some days or weeks after the first. The attention should not be so concentrated on the obvious that the less conspicuous is missed.

The history and examination of "the man who fell and hurt his arm" may serve to illustrate the preceding paragraphs. A twenty-five-year-old man enters the clinic complaining of pain in his left elbow of about four hours' duration. He states that while playing football he slipped and fell, landing with his arm under him. When he sat up, his elbow looked crooked and though there was not much pain he found he could not use the arm. His fellow-players pulled on his hand and something seemed to slip into place. As there was immediate improvement of function, the pa-

Classification and Diagnosis of Fractures

tient believed he was not seriously hurt and went home. The pain steadily increased, however, and the swelling became so marked that he decided to seek professional help. At no time has he noticed numbness or tingling in his fingers and he has been able to move them since the accident. There has been no previous injury to the arm and his general health has always been excellent. His job is that of a clerk in a dry goods store and he is certain it will be kept for him.

The examination shows a well-built young man in obvious pain but no apparent shock. His color is good and he is laughing and joking with his companions though he protects and supports his left elbow with his other hand. He removes his coat and shirt with considerable difficulty. Though there is marked swelling around the left elbow the axes of arm and forearm are similar to those of the opposite side and there is no visible deformity. The color of the skin is normal. Motions at the elbow are possible but are limited in extent. Flexion and extension of the forearm on the arm are about one-half the range of similar motions in the uninjured extremity and pronation and supination of the forearm about one-quarter. Wrist and finger motions are complete and painless. On gentle palpation it is found that the bony landmarks of the elbow-joint are in their normal positions. There is generalized tenderness around the entire elbow, but sharply localized tenderness over the radial head. Pressure on the radial heads makes voluntary pronation and supination almost impossible because of pain. Longitudinal compression of the forearm causes pain in the region of the radial head. The radial pulse is palpable and equal in strength to that on the uninjured side. No sensory changes are made out. There is no evidence of any other injury.

The tentative diagnosis is a reduced dislocation of the left elbow associated with a probable fracture of the radial head. X-ray examination is necessary for confirmation of the diagnosis.

18   Classification and Diagnosis of Fractures

Why is it necessary to waste time with a careful history and a thorough examination when x-ray pictures will demonstrate the fracture more accurately than by an other means? Unfortunately more and more emphasis is being placed on x-ray findings and less and less on clinical evaluation. In the first place x-ray machines are not always readily available, and the doctor must depend on his eyes and fingers for an immediate diagnosis. In the second place certain fractures, particularly of the carpal navicular, may not be demonstrable on x-ray plates taken shortly after the accident, and the immediate treatment must depend on the clinical picture. In the third place the accuracy of a reduction must frequently be checked at the time of manipulation by clinical means. Post-reduction films may not be available until the following day. Of course, the x-ray pictures are of inestimable value, but they should be used to support, not to supplant clinical observation and judgment. As has been said before, many fractures are compensation cases, accident cases, etc., and therefore medico-legal, and it should not be forgotten that x-ray films form an important part of the evidence.

Chapter 2

Bone Repair in Fractures

An understanding of the pathology of injury and the process of repair is necessary, both for the correct interpretation of the signs and symptoms resulting from the trauma, and for rational treatment. Some conception of the factors influencing the repair process is essential in the planning of definitive therapy.

When a bone breaks there is immediate bleeding from the torn periosteum, from the surrounding soft tissue and from the bone itself. The amount of this hemorrhage varies, obviously, with the size and number of blood vessels injured. A greenstick fracture is accompanied by a minute amount of extravasated blood; a comminuted, grossly displaced fracture may be surrounded by a pool of blood. Also as a result of the injury there is damage to the surrounding soft parts. This may consist of the death of a few cells or may mean extensive tearing of fascia, muscle, subcutaneous tissue and occasionally skin. Adjacent nerves may be injured and large blood vessels torn. The extent of the initial damage depends on the fracturing force; its subsequent course, however, is influenced by any secondary trauma which may occur.

The extravasated blood and the dead and damaged tissue act as an irritant and as a result there is locally an accumulation of inflammatory exudate at the fracture site with a local tissue infiltration of wandering cells. This process begins within a few minutes of the accident. Systemically a local inflammation with tissue death, if extensive, may manifest itself in a rise in temperature, an increased white cell count, a lowered hematocrit and evidences of shock.

Immediately following an injury there is usually a period of from twenty minutes to half an hour during which the nerve endings are insensitive, a period of tissue shock. During this time the muscles surrounding the fracture site are relaxed. After the immediate local tissue shock has subsided pain supervenes and the surrounding muscles go into protective spasm.

Repair processes begin almost as soon as injury occurs. They may be retarded or accelerated by various factors but the pattern is constant. First the extravasated blood clots and a fibrin network is formed in the clot. Fibroblasts grow in from the surrounding connective tissue; blood vessels bud into the mass and granulation tissue is formed. There is an absorption of calcium from the broken bone ends with a resulting concentration of calcium in the tissue fluids immediately surrounding the fracture site. Electrochemical examination at this time shows the tissue fluids to be slightly acid. As the circulation improves, the products of tissue death are removed by the blood stream. Also, with the improvement in the circulation, both blood and lymphatic, the acidity diminishes and the reaction of the tissue fluids becomes slightly alkaline. The calcium held in the tissue fluids is now deposited in the granulation tissue in rough, irregular trabeculæ, forming callus. With resorption and further deposition the trabeculæ become more dense and eventually new cortical bone is formed. Whether the deposition of calcium is brought about by the action of an osteogenetic cell, by an enzyme, or by some physico-chemical phenomenon is not a matter for discussion here. Conditions needed for bone healing are granulation tissue, calcium concentration in the immediate neighborhood and adequate circulation. How the calcium is actually deposited in the tissues to form bone is not known, nor has the chemical form of this calcium been identified.

Various factors influence or modify the process of repair. The first is the extent of the injury. If the damage to the bone is slight, as in a crack or buckling, the hemorrhage will be negligible and the resulting granulation tissue minimal.

If, on the other hand, the bone fragments are grossly displaced, the hemorrhage may be so great that the fluid is a block to repair and the formation of granulation tissue is much delayed. Multiple bone fragments, as seen in fractures caused by missiles, frequently heal surprisingly rapidly because the extent of bone surface increases the amount of calcium available in the surrounding tissues. The amount of soft tissue damage plays an important part in bone repair. Extensive stripping of the periosteum from the underlying bone tears the communicating vessels and interferes with the circulation. Injury to large vessels may compromise the circulatory status of the part not only by the tearing, thrombosis, or spasm of the vessels themselves but also by swelling and pressure from the resulting edema and/or hemorrhage. Injury to the muscles with massive lacerations and bruising will increase tissue necrosis and the extravasation of blood, resulting in further edema and later fibrosis. If the skin is injured the possible complication of infection is introduced.

The second factor modifying the repair process is the site of injury. A fracture through an area of bone which is surrounded by adequate soft tissue has a good blood supply and heals usually without difficulty. A fracture where there are few, if any, soft part attachments and an inadequate blood supply will heal slowly, if at all. For example, fractures of the neck of the femur and fractures of the proximal third of the carpal navicular are noted for their poor healing powers. Both regions are intracapsular and have no muscle attachments. Fractures of the intertrochanteric region of the femur, however, heal with abundant callus. A fracture into a joint will bleed into the joint but the blood will not clot unless there has been considerable associated soft tissue injury. Healing occurs with minimal callus formation because of the small amount of granulation tissue. A fracture through an epiphysis may result in growth disturbance because the injury may cause a premature ossification of the epiphyseal cartilage.

The type of bone, *i.e.*, cancellous or cortical, is also a factor in bone repair. The irregular trabeculæ of cancellous bone require little alteration from the embryonic type of trabeculæ in callus and healing proceeds rapidly. Because of its spongy texture, however, it is subject to change under stress for some time after the initial healing has occurred. The formation of cortical bone requires considerable rearrangement of the trabeculæ formed in callus and the healing process is much slower.

Of the systemic factors which influence bone healing, age plays a part only in the difference of healing between a child and an adult. The younger the child the more rapid will bone repair occur. After adolescence, age *per se* seems to have no marked influence. Systemic diseases, endocrine disturbances, conditions of the skeleton itself have little influence on the local repair processes unless there is a disease process involving the local area.

The factors so far discussed are outside the control of the doctor. Other factors, however, come directly into his sphere of influence. The first is secondary trauma. By this is meant the damage to the bone and to the surrounding tissues which is not caused by the original injury but results from careless transportation, rough examination and inadequate immediate splinting. The more extensive the soft part damage and the greater the circulatory embarrassment the slower will be the repair process.

The second is impaired circulation due not only to vascular damage but also to constricting bandages and splints, to dependency of the part, and to restricted muscle action. Adequate circulation, not only of blood but of lymph, is essential for the nourishment of the repair tissue. Improvement of circulation should be one of the chief concerns of the doctor. Other factors which have a direct effect on the healing of fractures and which are under the control of the doctor are interposition of soft tissue between the bone fragments, undue motion at the fracture site, and

Bone Repair in Fractures

separation of the bone ends. Muscle or periosteum caught between the fragments may act as a barrier to the formation of callus. Early recognition that this condition exists and prompt measures to correct it will prevent delayed healing. Inadequate immobilization of certain fractures in the shafts of long bones may result in fibrous union; but, on the other hand, prolonged splinting of fractures into a joint can lead to the formation of dense adhesions with marked impairment of function. Separation of the bone ends due to overpull or unwisely applied internal fixation can also result in delayed or non-union because of the inability of the callus formation to bridge the gap satisfactorily.

Chapter 3

Symptoms and Signs of Fractures

BEFORE discussing the principles of treatment let us attempt to translate the pathological and physiological changes described in the preceding chapter into terms of clinical significance. [When a patient receives a fracture he is aware of two symptoms, each of which is always present though in varying degree. The first is *pain*. This usually is instantaneous but may then disappear completely during the period of local tissue shock, leaving the patient aware only of a feeling of numbness. As the latent period passes off, pain may recur, to be sharply accentuated on every movement of the injured limb. Each motion of the unsplinted extremity drives the broken jagged bone ends into the surrounding tissues causing more bleeding, more swelling, more pressure, and more pain. The muscles of the limb contract spasmodically and as the muscles go into protective spasm with further shifting of the fragments the pain is increased, but can be relieved by the application of traction and firm splinting which will relax the spasm and tend to prevent motion at the fracture site. When there has been little displacement of the bones and when the fracture is incomplete the symptom of pain is much less prominent.] [Another manifestation of injury is that of *impairment of function*. The patient is aware that something is not right with the extremity and is conscious of the fact that he cannot use it.] This occurs even in cases where pain is not an outstanding characteristic. Frequently a patient will say that he "just knew there was something wrong with his arm" though he cannot explain why he felt that way. This is particularly true in children who after a fall will refuse to walk on a leg which shows no gross evidence of fracture

Symptoms and Signs of Fractures

and is apparently not painful. Careful examination and x-ray plates in two planes will frequently reveal in these cases a green-stick fracture of the tibia.

A broken bone presents certain signs as evidence of its existence. Each is not invariably present in every fracture, and some are present when no fracture exists. *Swelling*, though present in many other conditions, is one of the most constant signs of a fracture. When it occurs immediately after injury it is due to the bleeding from the bone and soft parts. It presents a circumscribed, sharply outlined appearance in contradistinction to the later indistinctly outlined swelling caused by the edematous infiltration. *Deformity* is a deviation from the normal anatomical structure. It is caused by displacement of the bony framework, as in a fracture or dislocation, but may also be caused by changes in configuration due to such conditions as neoplasm, tuberculosis, etc. Changes in shape, in length, in axis, in alignment and in rotation are all types of deformity and are caused by structural changes in bone or joint, most frequently by fracture or dislocation.

Ecchymosis, the discoloration of the skin due to the extravasation of blood, is very suggestive of a fracture when it appears at some distance from the painful area several days after injury. Ecchymosis which is visible immediately after the accident may be due to soft part injury alone or to such extensive tearing of tissue that the blood from the deep structures finds its way to the surface at once instead of draining along fascial planes. For example, ecchymosis seen in the front of an elbow immediately after a patient has received a severe fracture of the radial head indicates a torn joint capsule, lacerated brachialis fibers and damaged fascia which have allowed the blood from the broken bone to manifest itself under the skin. In a less severe injury the blood from the fractured radial head is held within the joint by the intact capsule as is evidenced by the clinical appearance of a hemarthrosis.

Symptoms and Signs of Fractures

Abnormal mobility can be manifested in three ways—the range of motion can be limited, the arc of motion can be altered, or there can be a false point of motion. For example, if an elbow can normally move from 30 to 185 degrees and after injury can move only from 80 to 130 degrees, there is definite limitation of motion. If, however, it can move from 50 to 205 degrees, the range of motion (155 degrees) is the same but the arc is different.

The signs so far described can all be seen. Other evidences of fracture can be elicited by palpation. The first of these is *direct tenderness*. This, however, can be misleading if there is a contusion or an abrasion at the fracture site for the tenderness may be due to the soft part damage caused by the blow. A more accurate sign of fracture is *indirect tenderness* which is produced by pressure in the long axis of the bone exerted at its two extremities. If there is a break in the continuity of the shaft such pressure will cause pain at the fracture site which is quite distinct from the pain of the injured soft parts. *Bony irregularity* can occasionally be felt when there is no visible deformity. The smooth contour of the cortex may be interrupted by a ridge or shelf of broken bone.

Two signs of fracture which are considered pathognomonic when they are present are *crepitus* and *false point of motion*. A word of warning should be inserted here that these two signs should not be elicited unless absolutely necessary because of the danger of causing further damage to the bone fragments and to the surrounding soft parts. Bony crepitus is the gritting sensation transmitted to the palpating fingers by the contact of the broken bone ends on each other. There are other forms of crepitus, that felt in certain types of tenosynovitis, in organizing hematomas, in cases of villous synovitis, but bony crepitus once felt is unmistakable. A false point of motion is that which occurs when there is a complete fracture of the shaft of a long

Symptoms and Signs of Fractures

bone, when there is obvious motion where no motion should be.

As has been said before, all these signs do not always occur in all fractures. Combinations of them are always present. For example, in the instance of a man with a reduced dislocation at the elbow and an undisplaced fracture of the radial head, pain and impaired function are present so both symptoms are observed. There is no gross deformity, no ecchymosis, but there is swelling and definite limitation of motion at the elbow. Palpation reveals tenderness over the head of the radius, and pressure on the forearm from wrist and elbow produces indirect tenderness at the same place. Crepitus and false point of motion are not present. Nevertheless the positive signs, *i.e.*, swelling, limitation of motion, direct and indirect tenderness, are sufficiently suggestive to warrant the diagnosis of fracture. A second case, that of an individual who has broken the shaft of a long bone, presents practically all the signs and symptoms described. Pain and loss of function are evident. There is gross deformity, *i.e.*, shortening of the leg and change in the axis of the bone. Ecchymosis is not visible, though it will be present in a few days. There is indirect tenderness, complete loss of motion of the extremity because of the lack of continuity of the shaft; there is a false point of motion easily visible and palpable. Crepitus in this case should be gently elicited because its absence is indicative of the interposition of soft parts which will not allow the bone ends to rub on each other.

The signs and symptoms so far discussed are all those of a fresh fracture. As time elapses the signs change in accordance with the changes going on within the extremity. At five days, for example, there will be less pain but still some impairment of function, depending upon the site of injury. If the deformity has not been corrected it will still be present; there will be considerable edematous swelling around the area. Ecchymosis in the dependent portion of the extremity will be visible. It will be less easy to palpate the bony irregularity because of the organizing hematoma around the bone ends. The range of motion will still be limited. Tenderness will be present but less sharply defined and indirect tenderness will also be present. There may still be abnormal mobility of the shaft but it will be less free because of the newly forming granulation tissue.

At five weeks the signs will have changed considerably. There will be no pain under ordinary circumstances and the limitation of function will be diminishing. The deformity will, of course, remain if it has not been corrected. The outline will be rounded, however, by the underlying callus. There will be no ecchymosis, for the discoloration will usually have disappeared by this time. The range of motion will have increased but probably will not have returned to normal. Tenderness and indirect tenderness will probably both be absent. Crepitus cannot be elicited and the only evidence of false point of motion will be a springy or an elastic sensation at the fracture site because the callus will be sufficiently formed to prevent motion of the bone ends. The callus may be palpable as a cylindrical or fusiform mass of tissue which feels dense and elastic.

Chapter 4

Principles of Treatment of Fractures

EMERGENCY TREATMENT OF FRACTURES

"Splint 'em where they lie!" is a time honored slogan and a most important one. To it should be added that every injury should be treated as a fracture until proved otherwise. Unnecessary emergency splinting never hurt anyone, but an unsplinted fracture is a potential danger. The secondary trauma caused by kindly but clumsy handling, ill planned transportation (*i.e.*, with the patient doubled up on the back seat of a sedan), overzealous examination, and no emergency splinting may cause far greater damage than the original accident.

A sixteen-year-old boy while playing sand-lot football was tackled and thrown in such a way that as he fell his leg was doubled over a stone. He felt immediate pain in his right thigh. His playmates lifted him to his feet but the leg crumpled under him and he fell again. He was dragged to the side of the field where it was some time before a passing motorist took him to his home. He was carried up three flights of stairs with the injured leg dangling and twisting in the arms of his bearers. A doctor was called who applied a wooden splint from hip barely to knee and ordered x-ray pictures. The family was so poor that a portable x-ray machine was not available, and the boy was carried down the three flights of stairs to the doctor's office where the x-ray films were made, then back up the stairs again. Twenty-four hours later the family was told that the boy had a broken femur and should be in the hospital. He was carried down the three flights of stairs again and taken in the back seat of a cab to the hospital. X-ray examination showed a long spiral fracture of the femur with nearly 3 inches overriding, both ends of the broken bone having pierced the surrounding muscles. An operation was necessary because of the damage to the soft parts and the interposition of the muscle.

Contrast this case with that of a slightly older boy who hurt his leg in an intercollegiate football game. He was allowed to lie where he fell on the field until the college physician could apply a Thomas splint. He was then taken from the field to the hospital. His x-ray films showed a complete fracture of the bone but in perfect anatomical position. There was little injury to the soft parts. The difference in healing time between these two cases was marked.

It seems to be instinctive for any layman witnessing an accident to lift the patient to a standing position, and unfortunately it is usually a layman and not a doctor who is first on the scene of the accident. Therefore widespread public education is being carried on by the Fracture Committee of the American College of Surgeons. Boy Scouts, firemen and police are being instructed in the application of splints.

The Thomas splint for fractures of the leg is the most efficient apparatus devised for temporary splinting and transportation. If one is not available, however, other means can be utilized for applying and maintaining traction in the long axis of the extremity and for holding the part immobilized until permanent treatment can be instituted. If there is no other way the leg can be pulled by doctor or layman against countertraction, with the pull maintained until the hospital is reached.

During the construction of a large bridge one of the workmen fell a distance of about 15 feet, landing with one leg twisted under him, the leg lying at right angles to the thigh. The foreman ran to him and, while another workman held the patient's shoulders, pulled on the leg, straightening it and maintaining constant pull while the man was rushed to the hospital by car. By the time he had reached the hospital the foreman had made an accurate reduction of the fracture.

Principles of Treatment of Fractures

Why should this be true? As we have seen in the preceding chapter, there is a latent period in practically all fractures before the muscles go into spasm. If traction can be applied during this period the length of the extremity may be maintained and overriding due to the pull of the muscles prevented. If the broken ends of the bone are allowed to move, the jagged ends may tear the surrounding fascia, muscles, and possibly nerves and blood-vessels. It is conceivable that a spike of bone may penetrate the skin, converting a closed fracture into one that is open.

So far nothing has been said about the effect of an unsplinted fracture on the general condition of the patient. Each move causes pain with its accompaniment of apprehension and fear, increases the shock, mental as well as physical, and so delays the return to normal. Treatment of the fracture should begin at the time of injury.

PERMANENT TREATMENT OF FRACTURES

After the patient has been brought to the hospital or to the doctor's office and the history, physical examination and x-ray pictures have been completed, the decision must be made as to the form of treatment best suited to the case. This choice does not depend primarily on the fracture. First an evaluation of the patient must be made. Is he dependable and coöperative? Can he be counted on to obey instructions or must some form of treatment be used which will protect him from himself? Is he economically independent? In other words, can he come to the hospital for needed care or must every effort be made to allow him to continue work while his fracture heals? What kind of work does he do? What is his general condition? Has he some respiratory or cardiac disease which will increase the danger of an anesthetic? Is he so old that it will be dangerous to keep him in bed? All these points must be kept in mind in the evaluation of the patient before definitive treatment is decided upon. There are times when the best treatment for the patient is not the best for the broken bone.

For example, an elderly but active woman came to the clinic for treatment of a badly broken wrist several days after the injury. Good reduction at that time might be possible, but it would necessitate a long period of immobilization of the wrist and hand with a protracted afterperiod of disability. It was wiser in that case to disregard the poor anatomy and bend every effort to regain useful function of the hand in as short a time as possible.

Next in importance to the evaluation of the patient is the form of treatment for which the doctor is best equipped. Is he working alone in a small town with limited assistance and equipment, or is he working in a large hospital with trained personnel and a smoothly running organization?

Also to be considered is his own experience and training—what type of treatment works best in his hands.

Finally comes the consideration of the type of fracture itself, its special problems and difficulties.

Reduction and Splints.—Keeping these considerations in mind we can now discuss the possible methods of treatment the doctor has at his disposal. First in general usefulness and therefore in importance is the method of closed reduction under an anesthetic, either general or local, followed by the application of some form of immobilization. Again it should be emphasized that the time for reduction is as soon after injury as possible in order to restore the broken bones to their normal position before the edema, granulation tissue, and muscle spasm have made this too difficult. The malposition of the broken bones may impair the circulation by direct pressure on the vessels, and thus increase the swelling which will persist until normal position of the fragments has been restored. "Wait until the swelling goes down" is very dangerous advice. In almost all cases anesthesia should be used for the reduction be-

Principles of Treatment of Fractures

cause it relaxes the muscle spasm, diminishes the amount of force necessary, and gives the operator time to do the thorough job which is practically impossible if the patient is conscious and suffering pain. The reduction should be done as gently as possible, not by any fixed set of maneuvers, but by those motions which will restore that particular broken bone to its normal position. This cannot be emphasized too strongly as each fracture is an individual problem and should be treated as such.

The splints which are applied after the reduction should be long enough to immobilize the fracture site adequately and yet not so long as to impede the motion of such joints as can be safely moved. If the patient is to be restored to activity as soon as possible it is important for him to maintain the function of the extremity insofar as it is consistent with the repair of the bone. For example, in a fracture of the wrist it is not only unnecessary but unwise to bring the splints down to the finger tips. The motion of the fingers in such cases is essential for the maintenance of the usefulness of the extremity.

Treatment by closed reduction and immobilization is satisfactory in many fractures. It is, however, of questionable use in those oblique fractures that tend to slip because of the muscle pull and the configuration of the bone ends. In such cases some form of continuous traction must be used.

Traction and Suspension.—Traction of various types has been of great value in fracture treatment from the time in the Middle Ages when a surgeon barber, who was called to see a French count suffering from a shattered leg, tied one end of a rope to the patient's foot and the other end to a stone which was allowed to hang over the end of the bed. It must be remembered that, although the words are commonly used together, traction and suspension are distinct entities. Each may be used without the other. Suspension of an extremity is useful for improving the circulation by position and for allowing freer motion in the suspended part than would be possible if the patient had to lift the extremity against gravity. Its use when coupled with traction is also to make the traction more efficient and to help in controlling the position of the fragments. Traction, on the other hand, regains length and helps to maintain the position obtained.

The same principle holds true for treatment by traction and suspension that holds in manipulative reduction, *i.e.*, that the reduction must be accomplished as soon as possible. In other words, the maximum weight needed to regain the length of the extremity should be applied at once and the position checked at frequent intervals by clinical and x-ray or fluoroscope examinations. When reduction is accomplished the weight should be reduced to the amount necessary to maintain the position. No doctor would consider reducing a fracture manually by a series of manipulations done at twenty-four-hour intervals. Why, therefore, should the attempt be made to reduce a fracture by traction by adding weights at daily intervals, in the hope of obtaining a reduction by the end of a week? The principles underlying both methods are the same. The earlier the reduction, the sooner the repair process can proceed unhindered.

Traction can be obtained in two ways: (1) By a pull on the skin by moleskin adhesive plaster or similar substances; or (2) by a direct pull on the bone by means of pins, tongs, or wires inserted into or through the bone. The skin is unable to stand a pull of much more than 10 pounds so this method is obviously limited in its use. It also is frequently uncomfortable and cannot be maintained over a long period because of irritation to the skin, particularly in old people. Skeletal traction, on the other hand, is efficient and apparently relatively comfortable. If properly applied it can be maintained for weeks. It is of importance to remember that the use of any form of skeletal traction must be accompanied by strict surgical technique to avoid possible infection.

Principles of Treatment of Fractures

A simple form of traction, called the Australian or Russell method, depends for its force on a double-pulley system and is effective and practical in certain fractures of femur and humerus (Fig. 2).

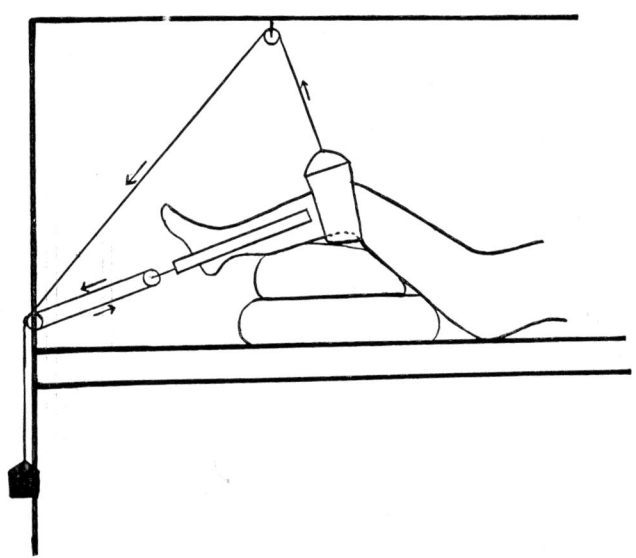

Fig. 2.—Russell traction.

The initial construction of the apparatus and the rigging-up of the patient in traction are but the first steps in the treatment, because a satisfactory result can be obtained only by constant care on the part of the doctors and nurses responsible for the patient. It is so easy for something to get out of place, for weights to rest on the floor or on projecting parts of the apparatus, for knots to catch in pulleys, for wrinkles to cause blisters. Traction, to be efficient, must be functioning twenty-four hours a day (Fig. 3).

It is frequently possible to couple the two methods so far described; that is, to apply traction for a period of time until full length has been obtained and then by manipulation slip the bone ends together. There is no reason why the use of one method should preclude the use of another.

The use of the traction suspension method necessarily means confinement in bed, usually in a hospital. Therefore, other methods have been devised to use the principle of fixed traction and allow the patient to be ambulatory. Pins inserted into the bone above and below the fracture are fastened to an external bar or bars after reduction has been obtained and hold the bone ends in position. Wires or pins

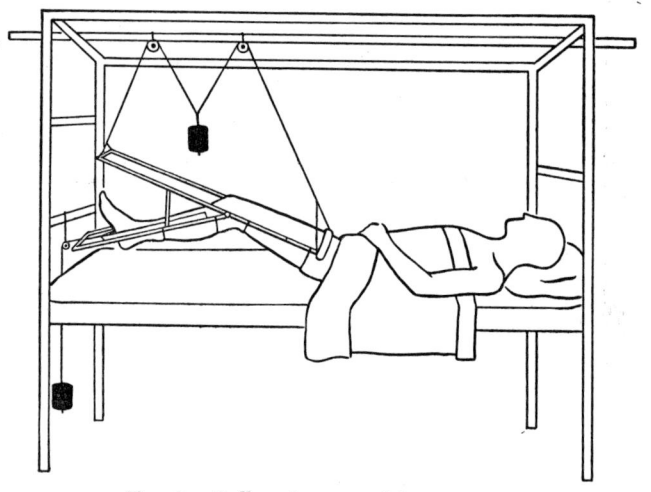

Fig. 3.—Balkan frame and leg traction.

passing through the bone can be incorporated in a plaster-of-Paris casing maintaining length. Aseptic precautions are necessary in the insertion of wires, for infection is a most unfortunate complication. The use of this principle has been satisfactorily applied to complicated fractures of the wrist, to oblique fractures of the forearm and to oblique or comminuted fractures of the leg.

Open Reduction of Fractures.—Operative interference is necessary in those cases where extensive internal hemor-

Principles of Treatment of Fractures

rhage or damage to a major blood vessel threatens the vitality of the extremity, where there is evidence of complete peripheral nerve injury and where there is interposition of soft tissue between the bone fragments. It is the wisest treatment when satisfactory position cannot be obtained or maintained by any other means.

Open operation with repair of the torn soft tissues and internal fixation of the bone fragments has for years been considered the method of choice for fractures of the patella and of the olecranon. The decision to operate should be made as soon as popssible. Delayed open reductions when the bone fragments are decalcified and callus has formed are difficult and not too satisfactory. Operations with internal fixation of the fracture should be performed as soon after injury as possible, certainly within a week or ten days or else postponed, if possible, until the bone has become recalcified.

Operative reduction with internal fixation as a method of choice for fractures other than of the patella and the olecranon is becoming an accepted form of treatment. The underlying principle is that of an internal splint which permits the rapid return of muscle and joint action while maintaining rigid fixation of the bone. Steel plates and screws, intramedullary pins, and metal bands are used for this purpose. The dangers of the method are obvious for the bruised and injured tissues resulting from the initial injury provide an admirable medium for bacterial growth and an osteomyelitis as a result of operation is a disaster. Adequate technique, skilled assistants, tested equipment and a smoothly running organization are absolutely essential for the success of the operative method. If rigid internal fixation has been achieved, external splinting for more than a few days defeats the purpose of the operation.

Open or Compound Fractures.—Immediate operation for the surgical cleansing of the wound is the accepted treatment for all fractures with a communicating wound in the

38 Principles of Treatment of Fractures

skin. This is still true in spite of the many antibiotics now available. These cases are all contaminated by the initial trauma, and the sooner they are surgically cleansed the less danger there is that infection will supervene. They should be considered as much of an emergency as an acute appendix.

At operation all dead and dying tissue should be removed by sharp dissection beginning at the skin margins. The wound should be enlarged to afford adequate exposure and allow the washing out of dirt and debris by thorough irrigation with normal saline or sterile water. Chemical disinfectants like iodine should never be used because of their deleterious action on the living cells. If particles of dirt cannot be washed out they must be excised. The irrigation and debridement should proceed into the depths of the wound layer by layer with frequent changes of gloves and instruments in order that contamination will not be carried into the depths. Small bone fragments with no soft tissue attachments may be removed, but it is wise to leave all fragments that have a chance of survival.

After the wound has been made as surgically clean as possible the fracture can be treated as the surgeon sees fit. The decision to close the wound should be made by experienced surgeons, based on the consideration of the length of time elapsed since injury, the type of trauma and the amount of contamination and tissue damage. If the case is seen within a couple of hours after the accident, if the open fracture was caused by a sharp object like an axe or a saw and the soft tissue damage was minimal, the wound might safely be closed. It is usually wiser to leave it open, covered, but not packed, with fine meshed gauze and to do a delayed closure at five days.

The administration of penicillin and other bacteriostatic agents is a valuable aid to control infection but in no way replaces careful surgery. Before a patient with an open fracture reaches the operating room, however, certain things

Principles of Treatment of Fractures

must be done. When the case is first seen the wound should be immediately covered by a sterile dressing. No attempt at cleansing should be made at the time, for it can be carried out more quickly and carefully and with less shock to the patient when he is under an anesthetic. It may be considered wise not to pull projecting bone fragments back into the wound because of the danger of spreading the contamination. The extremity should be splinted in such cases without traction. However, the present teaching is that the danger of spreading the contamination is less than the harm done by uncontrolled motion of the bone fragments and emergency traction is usually advised. The general condition of the patient must be watched and supportive measures, such as morphine, heat, intravenous fluids, etc., given if necessary. Tetanus antitoxin or toxoid booster should be given in all cases of open fracture. Roentgenograms are of great assistance to the surgeon and should be taken as soon as possible.

The shorter the interval between injury and operation, the better will be the results.

REHABILITATION

Rehabilitation is "the restoration to useful activity of individuals who have been wounded so as to suffer from physical or emotional disability, such restoration including treatment of the disability and training to fit the individual for occupation in industry." (Dorland, 22nd Ed.) In simpler terms it means making the patient well again in body and in mind. It involves many agencies and has become a complicated and elaborate process since World War II. It should start from the time of injury and carry through until the patient has reached the maximum return of his capabilities. The doctor who is in charge of the care of the injury is responsible for the ultimate result and should use all the means available in his community to attain the best result possible. It is not enough to have achieved a solidly healed fracture in good position—the patient must be able to use the extremity and be ready to return to his place in the community both physically and mentally.

Reassurance of the patient should start immediately and "compensationitis" nipped in the bud. Active motion of every joint that can safely be moved should be encouraged from the beginning. It is far easier to keep joints moving than to mobilize stiffened extremities. Stiff fingers and toes are an unnecessary handicap.

Exercises for the uninjured parts of the body should be started early and kept up. Even if a patient is in a plaster spica or a Thomas splint the rest of his muscles can and should move.

Heat, massage, whirlpool baths and other physical aids are useful but do not take the place either psychologically or physically of what the patient does for himself. Gym classes and games, where the patient forgets his injured extremity, all help to make him active and well. Even the old ladies with broken hips should be out of bed as soon as possible and entering into ward activities. They should not be allowed to become mental invalids.

After the patient has left the hospital or after his splints or casing have been removed the doctor's responsibility is not finished. The weakened muscles must be strengthened, the stiffened joints loosened, and the inevitable discouragement combatted. Physical therapy with supervised active exercise is of great help, but the patient must not be allowed to rely on other peoples' efforts. Diathermy three times a week will not take the place of a series of exercises done three or four times a day at home.

Occupational therapy plays an important part in any rehabilitation program. This may tax the doctor's ingenuity and inventive powers but is well worth the effort. Weaving, knitting, wood-carving, jig-saw work, and similar occupations have the advantage of focusing the attention of the patient on what he is making rather than on the action of his injured limb, with the result that the coördination is far better. A patient is much more likely to play nine holes of golf five times a week when prescribed by his doctor than to walk the same distance with no objective. The walk is boring but golf is interesting. Occupational therapy can be carried on in the home several hours a day and helps the patient to return to his normal activities faster than almost any other form of treatment.

If it is possible to get the patient back to work, even at a different job for a while, it is most important to do so. The work habit is easily lost if convalescence is prolonged and is hard to regain. Sitting around the house watching television strengthens neither mind nor body.

Vocational guidance and vocational training where they are available are of great assistance where the injuries are such that the patient is unable to return to his previous occupation. The wise doctor will know the facilities afforded by his community or where they can be obtained.

Follow-up.—No discussion of fracture treatment is complete without some mention of follow-up evaluation. Changes due to epiphyseal or circulatory alterations may occur in joints or bones that do not become evident for two, three or even five years after injury. An apparently good result at three months may become a mediocre or poor one at three years, and a discouraging case at a few weeks may eventually prove most satisfactory. Anatomical, functional and economic evaluations compared with x-ray findings provide a yardstick by which to measure the efficacy of different methods of treatment. Analysis of results then becomes factual and not impressionistic. The follow-up clinic is one of the most important features of a fracture service as it affords an objective analysis of late results.

Chapter 5

Details of Technique in Treatment of Fractures

THE APPLICATION OF EMERGENCY SPLINTS

A THOMAS splint (Fig. 4) can be simply and quickly applied by an individual alone if he has had practice. As

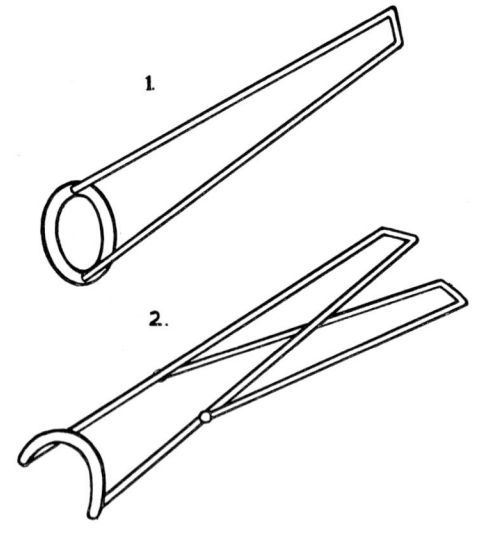

FIG. 4.—1, Emergency splint; 2, half-ring splint with footpiece for suspension.

the patient lies on the ground the bandage to be used for traction should first be tied around the ankle with the shoe left in place and adequate padding placed between the tie and the extremity. Various knots can be used for this purpose; one of the simplest is shown in the illustration (Fig. 5). With the bandage or rope in place traction can be exerted by direct pull on the rope and the leg straightened out. The pull should not be relaxed at any time. The ring of the Thomas splint can then be slipped over the foot and

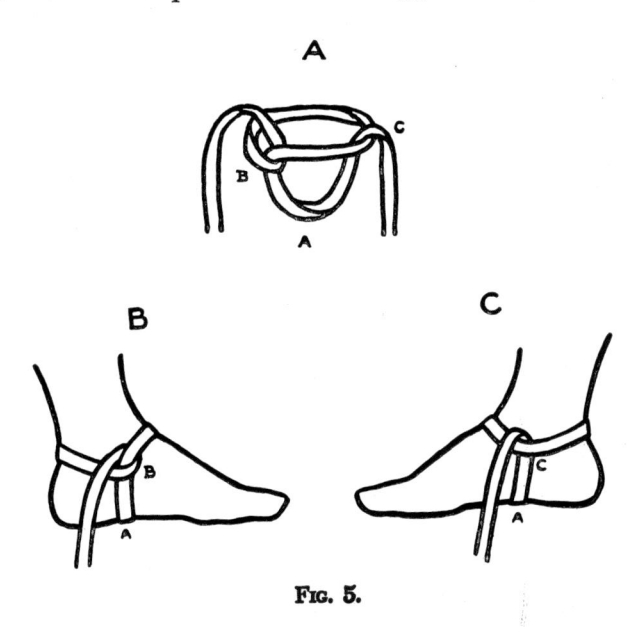

Fig. 5.

the splint gently pushed up the leg until the ring rests against the ischial tuberosity. Care must be taken in an unconscious patient to avoid pressure against the scrotum or labium. The two ends of the traction rope can then be tied at the end of the splint and traction increased by twisting the rope with a stick, the so-called "Spanish windlass" method. A snug bandage tied around both the extremity and the splint at the mid-thigh, above and below the knee, and in the middle of the leg, will hold the limb firmly in place and the patient can be transported with relative comfort. Care must be taken not to allow the patient's heel to rest on mattress or stretcher. This can be avoided by supporting the end of the splint on a folded pillow or a similar rest. If a Thomas splint must remain in place for any length of time the circulation of the foot must be carefully watched

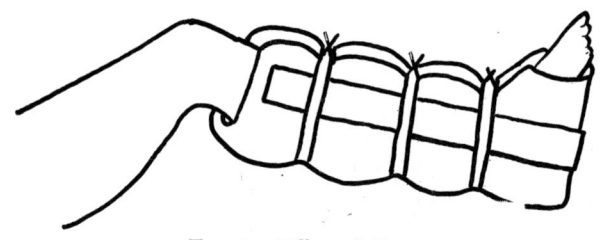

Fig. 6.—Pillow Splint.

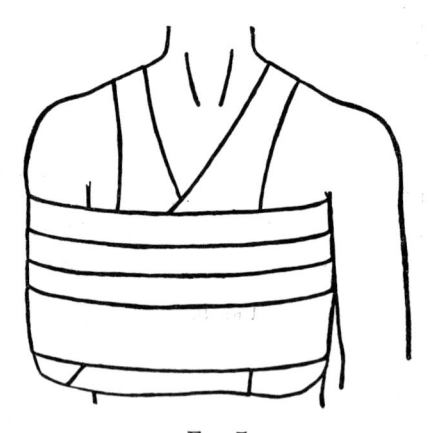

Fig. 7.

and all points of pressure carefully padded to avoid subsequent skin breakdown.

The Tobruk splint evolved by the British in World War II is a useful modification of the emergency Thomas splint if the patient has to be transported for a considerable distance. After the leg has been placed in the splint and traction applied (preferably by longitudinal adhesive strips)

Technique in Treatment of Fractures

plaster-of-Paris bandages are wrapped around the extremity and the bars of the splint, holding the leg more firmly than by ordinary bandage. The outer side of the ring should be well-padded to hold it away from the greater trochanter.

If a Thomas splint is not available the doctor should be able to improvise from the material at hand a means of immobilization. Ironing boards, shelves, even cellar doors can be utilized. A child with a fractured femur was safely and comfortably transported to a hospital on a bookshelf. Traction was applied by a bandage tied around the ankles

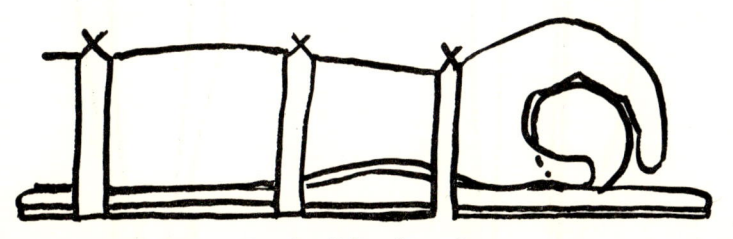

Fig. 8.—Splint for wrist.

and passed snugly around the back of the board (which was slightly longer than the patient) to end in a loop under the child's shoulders.

For injuries involving the lower leg and ankle padded board splints may be used. If there is gross deformity a pillow bandaged snugly around the leg and foot and reinforced by wooden strips if available is a safe and relatively comfortable method of emergency immobilization (Fig. 6).

Suspected dislocations of the shoulder and fractures of the humeral shaft can be well protected by means of a sling with a swathe around arm and body (Fig. 7). Padded wooden splints are excellent for the emergency care of injuries to the forearm, wrist, or hand with a roller bandage, a ball or an inverted cup under the palm to hold the hand and fingers in a slight curve. Magazines make good splints for forearm and wrist fractures (Fig. 8).

ADHESIVE STRAPPING

The use of adhesive plaster for a support for an injured joint is very common. It can also be used in fracture cases after the removal of the plaster-of-Paris appliance and before the injured part has regained full strength. If the adhe-

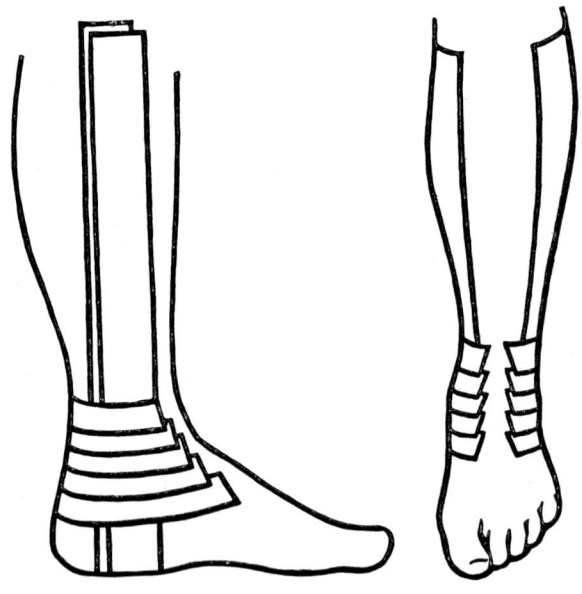

Fig. 9.—Ankle strapping.

sive plaster is to be applied directly to the skin the surface should be shaved and cleaned. Tincture of benzoin applied directly on the surface to be strapped will protect the skin from irritation and make the adhesive plaster stick better. There are many different forms of ankle strapping, most of them good. A simple type, as shown in the illustration, consists of two 2-inch strips extending from the outer side of the knee around the instep to the inner side of the knee and held in place by narrower strips around the ankle

Technique in Treatment of Fractures

(Fig. 9). The foot should be at right angles to the leg and either in mid-position or slight inversion. No strapping of an ankle should be circumferential because of the danger of swelling of the dependent part. Strapping should

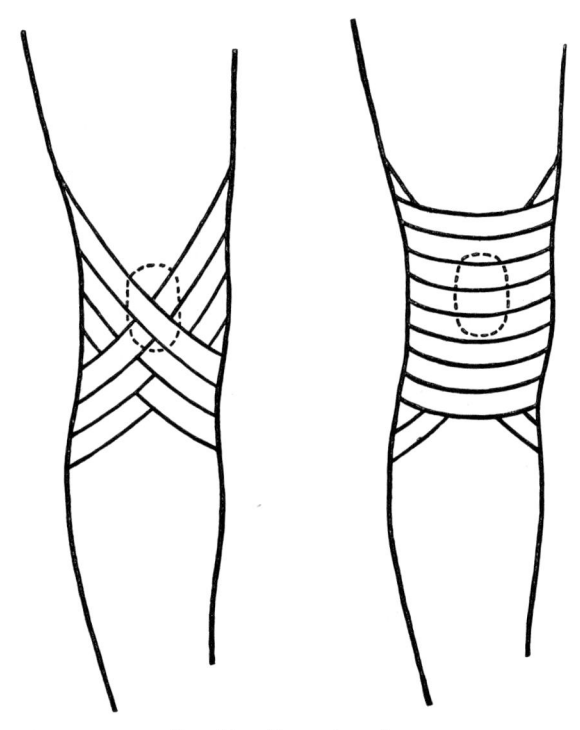

FIG. 10.—Knee strapping.

be put on with considerable firmness, not just laid on. Satisfactory strapping for the knee is shown in the illustration (Fig. 10). Strapping for the chest should always go beyond the midline, both in front and in back, otherwise it is ineffectual. It is difficult to strap a woman's chest with adhesive plaster directly applied to the skin. A circumferential flannel binder held up by shoulder straps and then covered by

4-inch adhesive applied securely gives a very satisfactory support. This is also more comfortable for men with hairy chests. A support for the wrist can be made by the use of snug-fitting stockinette wrapped firmly with adhesive plaster. To make this removable it can be split, bound with

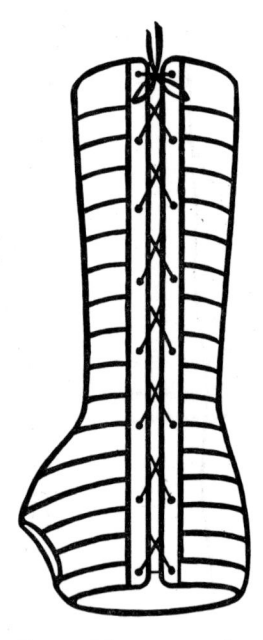

FIG. 11.—Removable support for the wrist.

adhesive, and laced with a shoelace or tape through holes punched in the edge (Fig. 11). Similar removable dressings can be made for an ankle.

PLASTER-OF-PARIS SPLINTS AND CASINGS

It is not within the scope of this book to describe all the types of plaster-of-Paris dressings. Each surgeon has his own techniques, but certain hints in the use of this material

Technique in Treatment of Fractures 49

may be found helpful. The making of a splint is a simple procedure if the commercially prepared plaster-of-Paris bandages are used. The required length, measured on the

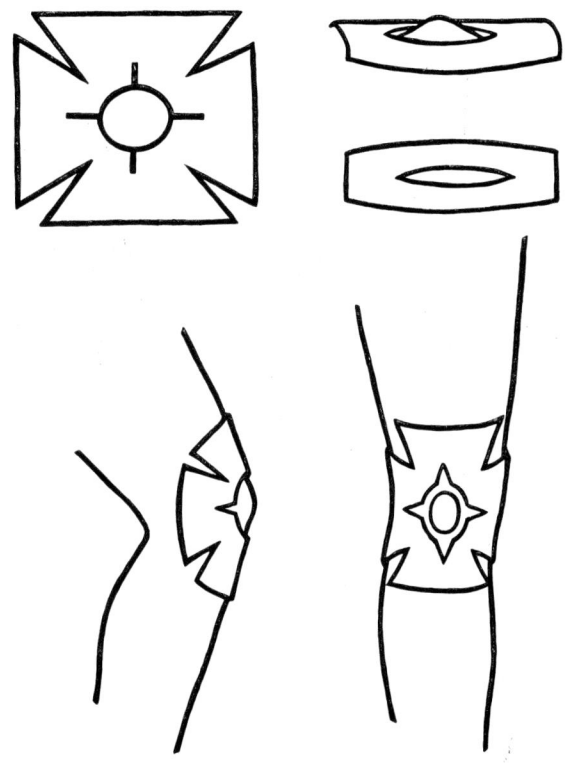

Fig. 12.—Types of felt padding.

uninjured extremity, is ascertained and the dry bandage unrolled back and forth until the desired number of layers is reached. It is then dipped in a pail or basin of warm water, for the length of time necessary for the particular make of bandage, and spread out on a smooth flat surface. Care should be taken to rub the wet plaster thoroughly in order that the gauze be completely impregnated before applying it to the patient. The plaster may be covered by a layer of Canton flannel or stockinette to protect the skin. The roll of prepared plaster may be soaked before it is unrolled and the layers made from the wet plaster. If this method is used

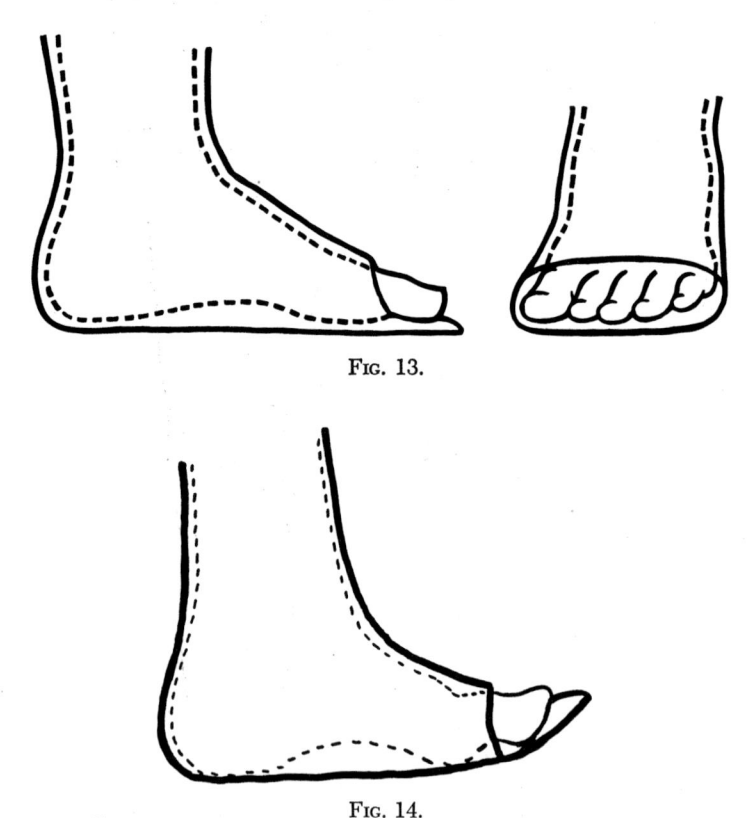

Fig. 13.

Fig. 14.

each layer must be rubbed in as it is laid down. The wet splint is then bandaged firmly in place on the extremity and allowed to dry. When the plaster has hardened the bandages should be cut off as the dampness may cause the gauze to shrink and cut into the skin. The splint should always

Technique in Treatment of Fractures

be rebandaged before the patient is permitted to leave. Great care should be taken not to allow any motion while the plaster is setting, otherwise a "hinged" splint or casing will result.

If padding is used over bony prominences under a circular plaster it should be so cut that is surrounds the prominence instead of pressing directly upon it (Fig. 12). The plaster should be applied smoothly and constantly rubbed in with careful molding to the contours of the part. Plaster casings should always be so applied that they extend far enough not to cut into the soft parts as in mid-calf or mid-forearm and yet not so far as to interfere with motion in the adjacent joints. A gauntlet for a wrist should extend from the mid-palmar crease to about 1 inch below the elbow. A plaster boot should extend from the toes to about 1 inch below the knee. It is more comfortable for the patient if any plaster which includes the foot is carried to a little beyond the tip of the toes on the plantar surface and to the metatarsophalangeal joints on the dorsal (Fig. 13). This gives room for motion of the toes and supports them on the plantar surface, thereby preventing cutting at the edge of the plaster. Care must be taken not to dorsiflex the toes as clawing may result with considerable disability (Fig. 14). It is frequently wiser to stop the plaster sole at the metatarsal heads to allow flexion of the toes. Leg casings which do not include the foot tend to slip up and down. This can be remedied by placing two long strips of adhesive plaster on the skin of the medial and lateral aspects of the extremity. The plaster-of-Paris is then applied over the strips, the ends of which are turned back and incorporated in the casing. Care must be taken to get the plaster high enough. All splints and casings should have smooth edges to avoid irritation of the skin.

Any casing that is applied for the immobilization of a recently reduced fracture or of an injury likely to cause further swelling must be split for its entire length. Failure to observe this precaution may result in disastrous impairment of the circulation. If for any reason it is felt unwise to split the plaster-of-Paris the patient should be kept under constant observation until the danger of further swelling is over.

Various motor-driven saws and knives have been invented to aid in the removal of plaster jackets, spicas, and extremity casings. However, these are not always available. The most useful and the most foolproof instrument is the two-handled plaster-cutting instrument with a cutting, saw-tooth upper blade and a dull, flat lower blade to slip between the plaster and the skin. An old scalpel or a razor blade is helpful in cutting around corners but must be used with caution. Hydrogen peroxide will soften the plaster somewhat, but usually patience and persistence applied to the plaster-cutting instrument will suffice to remove any casing.

ASPIRATION OF JOINTS

Aspiration of a joint is a very valuable therapeutic measure in cases where fractures into the joint have caused a hemarthrosis with resulting pain and disability. It may be safely carried out if done under strict surgical precautions. The joint to be aspirated should be shaved, cleaned and prepared as for an operation. The operator should use sterile gloves. At the site chosen for the insertion of the needle a small bleb is made in the skin with novocaine. An incision is made in the bleb with a sharp-pointed scalpel so that skin contamination is not carried down into the depths by the aspirating needle. The needle used for skin injection is discarded, a second needle longer than the first is inserted, and the novocaine is injected down to and into the capsule of the joint. After a minute or two to allow the novocaine to take effect, an aspirating needle of large bore is inserted into the joint cavity and the fluid removed. An elbow joint may be aspirated on the postero-lateral

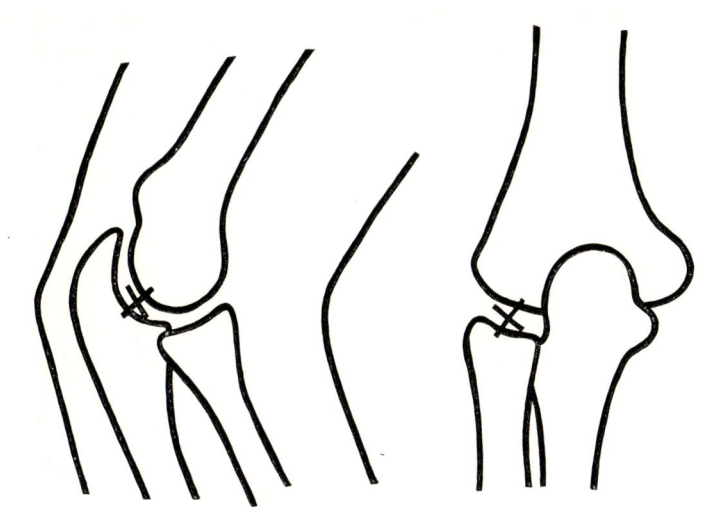

Fig. 15.—Site for aspiration of the elbow joint.

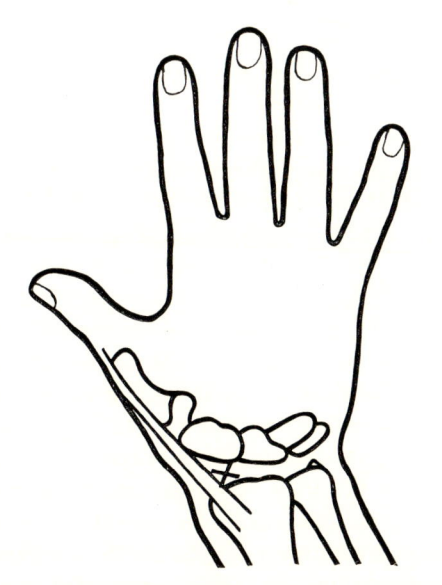

Fig. 16.—Site for aspiration of the wrist joint.

aspect in the mid-point of the triangle formed by the tip of the olecranon, the lateral epicondyle and the radial head (Fig. 15). The wrist joint may be aspirated in the dorsal surface just medial to the tendon of the extensor longus pollicis (Fig. 16). The knee may be aspirated on either side of the patella at its upper or at its lower margin (Fig. 17). The ankle may be aspirated at a point on the anterolateral aspect about 2.5 cm. cephalad to the tip of the fibula and 1 cm. medial.

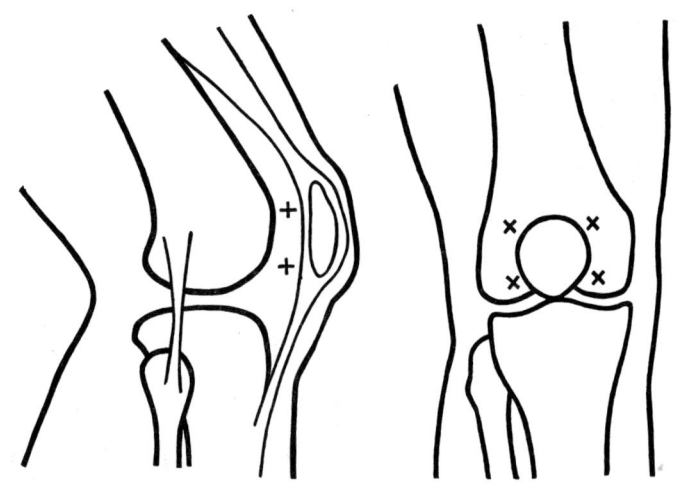

Fig. 17.—Sites for aspiration of the knee joint.

LOCAL ANESTHESIA FOR REDUCTION

The technique for the injection of novocaine for the reduction of a fracture is similar to that used in aspirations and similar precautions should be observed. The site for injection should be directly over the fracture. The injecting needle, inserted after the skin nick, should go directly into the hematoma which always surrounds the bone ends in the first few hours after injury. Ten to 15 cc. of a 1 or 2 per cent solution of novocaine should then be injected into the hema-

Technique in Treatment of Fractures 55

toma. It is important to allow five or ten minutes to elapse after the injection of the novocaine before any manipulation of the fracture is attempted. Failure to do this causes considerable pain to the patient and may diminish the efficacy of the anesthesia.

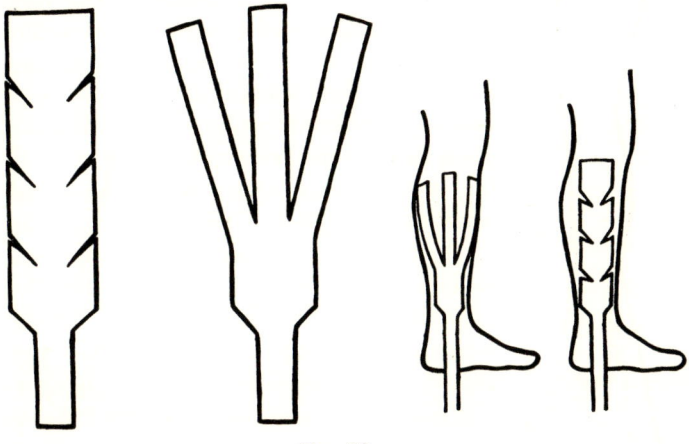

Fig. 18.

TRACTION SUSPENSION APPARATUS

There are many different types of frames in use, each with its own peculiarities. However, there are certain details which are common to them all. In setting up a frame for use with skin traction it is better to apply the adhesive material to the skin before the rest of the apparatus is assembled. That allows time for the plaster or flannel to become firmly adherent to the skin before the weight is attached to it. The adhesive plaster must be absolutely smooth, as a wrinkle will cause an irritation or blister in the skin. To make it fit it should be cut in such a way as not to weaken its tensile strength (Fig. 18). It should not press on any bony prominences but the spreader, on the other hand, should not be so much wider than the extremity that it will tend to strip the adhesive upward (Fig. 19). To hold the adhesive firmly to the skin an elastic bandage should be snugly and smoothly applied. The upper inch of plaster, however, should remain exposed to view so that a glance will show if it is beginning to slip.

If skeletal traction is preferred the wire should be introduced through a nick in the skin under strict aseptic technique. Either a motor drill or a hand drill can be used and any number of gadgets have been devised to hold the wire rigid as it goes into the bone. The skin should be cut at the point of emergence as well as at the point of entrance so that there is no undue tension at the skin edge. A small cotton collodion dressing is all that is needed for the wound. It should be remembered that wire should always be inserted from the dangerous side, *i.e.*, where there are structures to be avoided, because the point can be placed in the bone either by direct vision or blunt dissection. The point of emergence, however, is less controllable. For example, at the elbow the wire should be inserted at the medial aspect of the olecranon as the ulnar nerve can thus be avoided. At the lower end of the femur the medial side is again the side of choice for the insertion of the wire so that there will be no danger of the emerging point entering the adductor canal (Hunter's canal).

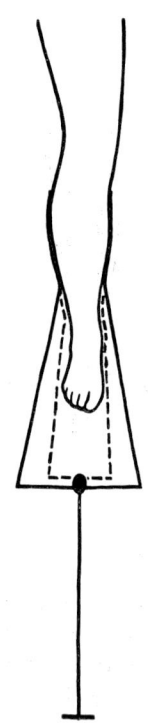

Fig. 19.—Solid line shows incorrect spreader.

After either form of traction has been applied to the extremity, the apparatus must be so lined up that the direction of pull is parallel to the axis of support. The traction rope should be sufficiently short so that there is no danger of the weights resting on the floor or on a bar of the bed. Ropes must run freely through the pulleys. Supporting swathes must be smooth and maintain an even pressure. If much weight is being used, shock blocks to counteract the pull will help to prevent the patient from being pulled out of bed. For instance, if there is great traction on the lower extremity the foot of the bed should be elevated by shock blocks. If there is considerable traction on the arm, the side of the bed should be raised to keep the patient from being pulled too near the edge.

Some form of appliance should be used to prevent footdrap. An adhesive plaster sole attached by a rope through a pulley to a light weight will work very satisfactorily.

No matter what type of rope is used for rigging up the apparatus all knots should be bound with adhesive tape to prevent slipping or fraying. The sudden collapse of suspension is frightening to the patient and may have a disastrous effect on the fracture.

When it is desired to remove the wire, one end can be cut flush with the skin by a pair of wire cutters. The tip is then painted with iodine or alcohol and the remaining end grasped by a clamp and pulled steadily. No anesthesia is necessary. If the wire has been in place for some time it is usually extracted with very little effort.

Chapter 6

Accident Ward Procedure

In many of the smaller hospitals internes fresh from medical school are frequently put into the accident room with little or no instruction or advice as to how to handle the problems they will meet. In many places they have no residents to call on for immediate help, and they quite naturally hesitate to ask an attending surgeon for assistance in what may be a minor problem. It is to try to help such men and women that this chapter is written.

Much has been written about the treatment at the site of accident; and there are many volumes describing the definitive procedures to be instituted after the diagnosis and extent of the injuries have been ascertained; but there is a gap between the initial and the definitive treatment, that period where the patient is first seen in the accident room, which is rarely if ever mentioned. It is a most important period, for much harm can be done and lives can be lost by inexperienced though well meaning individuals.

It should always be remembered that to many patients their experience in the accident ward is their first introduction to the hospital, and this first impression can be of importance. Courtesy, gentleness, and consideration on the part of everyone caring for the patient should be as much a part of the treatment as emergency splints. To the patient his cut or bruise is as important to him as it is insignificant to the interne, who may have had to get out of bed to see it. Nevertheless a little kindness on the part of the doctor is definitely in order. Of course it is annoying to be called at 2 A.M. to care for an injury that happened several hours before, and it is hard to avoid being irritable, but it pays off in improved public relations.

Accident Ward Procedure

When a seriously injured patient is brought into the hospital the first and most important thing to do is to be sure that breathing is not embarrassed, that the airway is clear. There are times when an emergency tracheotomy is a lifesaving measure. Of equal importance is the control of gross hemorrhage, if it has not already been done at the site of accident. A firm pressure dressing will slow down all except major arterial bleeding.

After these two obvious precautions have been observed the wise interne will decide what help he will need, a laboratory technician for blood grouping and cross matching, an x-ray technician for roentgenograms, and probably an attending surgeon. If the accident has occurred at night it is quite possible that none of these individuals is in the hospital, and it will save time if they can be alerted.

If there are evidences of shock, intravenous fluids should be started, plasma expanders or plasma, until such time as whole blood is available. Obvious fractured extremities should be splinted if that has not already been done at the site of the accident. There seems to be a widespread feeling that once a patient is within the walls of a hospital he is *ipso facto* immune from any further trauma, and temporary splinting is unnecessary. Unfortunately the patient has to be moved, to be examined, to be x-rayed, to be transferred to bed or operating room table; and broken bones must be protected. Obviously the less he is moved the better, but emergency splinting is still essential.

A gentle and rapid examination of the patient must be done to ascertain the extent of the injuries. Although it may take a few extra minutes, the findings should be written down at once. If there are two or three patients in the accident ward at the same time it is all too easy to be confused if the examinations are written up several hours later. In cases of head injury changes in the neurological findings are of extreme importance, and it is not safe to trust to memory, especially if there are several people hurt.

Above all things use your head. Common sense is a most valuable commodity, especially in an emergency, and a quiet, unhurried manner will often quiet the confusion of milling relatives, police and helpful friends.

Those injuries which present an immediate threat to life are of first concern. An open fracture of the femoral shaft may be a dramatic and apparently urgent matter, but if it is accompanied by a ruptured spleen or a crushed chest it becomes of secondary importance. The wound can be debrided during the same anesthesia that is used for the laparotomy if the plan of attack has been carefully worked out. With the use of antibiotics debridement can be delayed for twenty-four to forty-eight hours, if the life of the patient demands it.

Superficial lacerations rarely if ever threaten life, and yet there is an almost irresistible urge on the part of most internes to suture any and all cuts before doing anything else. Lacerations can wait twenty-four hours if necessary. They should, of course, be carefully evaluated to make sure that there are no cut tendons or broken bones beneath. If the patient is going to be given an anesthetic for the reduction of a fracture or for an operative procedure, the various superficial wounds can be better sutured at the same time with far less discomfort to the patient.

Immunization against tetanus must be carried out in all open fractures, all gunshot wounds, and all lacerations that have occurred out of doors. Most children and all men and women who have been in the armed services have received tetanus toxoid and need therefore only have booster shots, if the previous injection has been within four years. (Some authorities say that a longer period is still safe.) The tetanus antitoxin must always be preceded by a skin test. If this is positive, advice should be asked before proceeding with the injection.

Part II. The Upper Extremity

Chapter 7

Injuries to the Shoulder Girdle

FRACTURES OF THE CLAVICLE

Occurrence.—A common form of injury, particularly in children, this fracture is usually due to the indirect trauma of a fall on the outstretched arm or on the shoulder, less frequently to a direct blow.

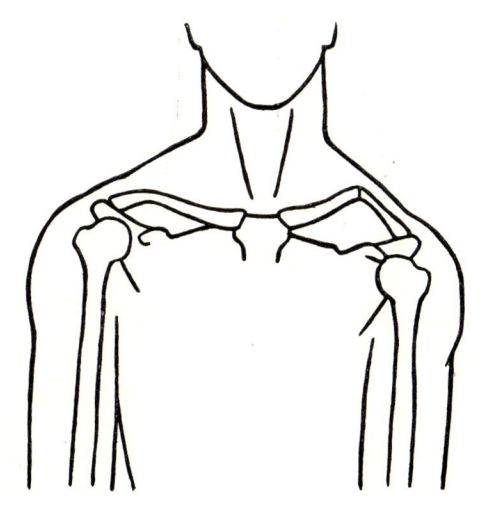

Fig. 20.

Displacement.—The clavicle acts as the anterior supporting strut to the shoulder. Therefore when the fracture occurs in the shaft at the most frequent site of break, *i.e.*, the junction of the middle and outer thirds where the two curves of the bone unite, the shoulder tends to droop downward, forward, and medially (Fig. 20). Displacement of the fragments is caused by the fracturing force and by the weight of the upper extremity. There may be overriding

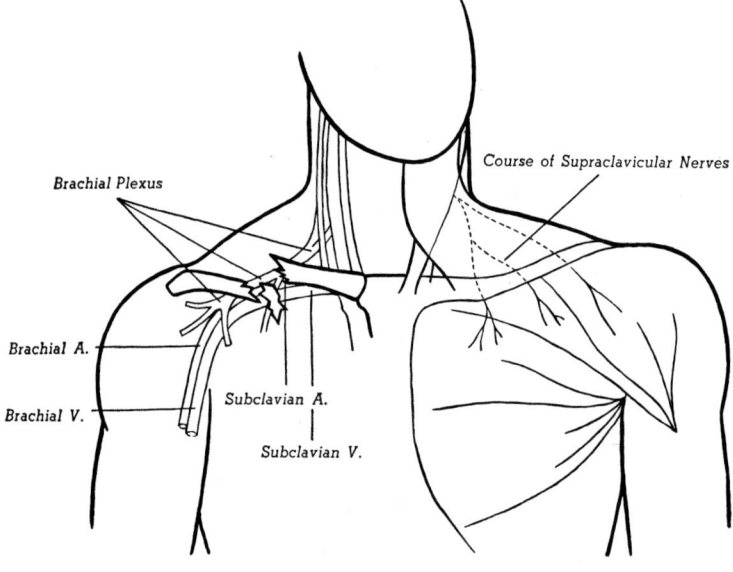

Fig. 21.

or, especially in the incomplete fractures of childhood, angulation with the apex of the angle pointing upward (Fig. 20). Fractures in the outer third may show no displacement if the coraco-clavicular (conoid and trapezoid) ligaments are intact, or may be displaced upward simulating an acromio-clavicular dislocation (*q.v.*). Injuries at the inner third rarely show displacement due to the restraining influence of the costo-clavicular (rhomboid) ligament.

Diagnosis.—Due to its subcutaneous position the clavicle is easily palpated throughout its extent and the diagnosis of

Injuries to Shoulder Girdle

fracture is usually easy. Irregularity of bony contour, localized tenderness and disability should be sufficient to suggest such an injury. X-ray pictures are always essential to confirm the clinical findings.

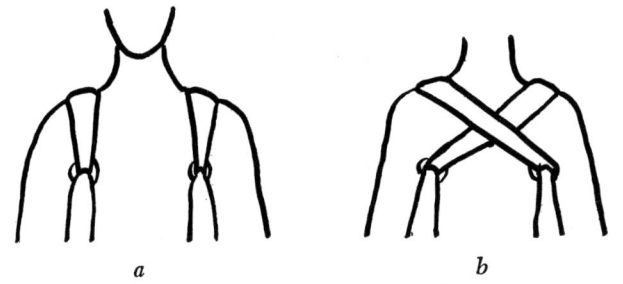

Fig. 22.—Figure-of-eight; *a*, anterior; *b*, posterior.

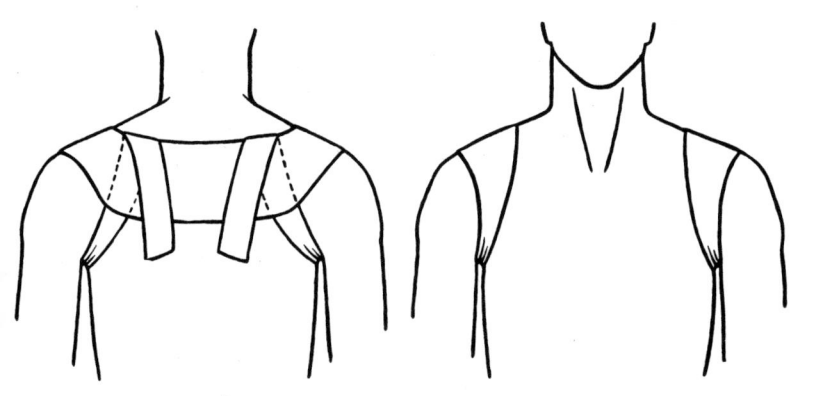

Fig. 23.

Pathology.—Swelling and ecchymosis may be minimal or moderate, depending on the amount of displacement of the fragments with the resultant tearing of the soft parts. Because of the close relationship of the platysma to the bone the muscle fibers are occasionally pierced by a projecting fragment and may become interposed between the broken ends. Injury to the supraclavicular nerves may occur and

64 Injuries to Shoulder Girdle

less frequently injury to the underlying brachial plexus (Fig. 21). The latter is most often associated with a direct blow on the clavicle depressing the fragments. More rarely damage to the subclavian vessels has been reported.

Treatment.—Fractures in children can be satisfactorily treated with figure-of-eight flannel bandage around the shoulders and crossing at the back (Fig. 22). In older children a plaster-of-Paris double L shoulder splint carefully molded and well padded in the axillae holds the fracture more securely (Fig. 23). The patient should be seen frequently to insure maintenance of the bandage or splint and to watch for irritation and pressure under the arms. The bandage or splint should be maintained for three weeks, and the child encouraged to use the arm during that period.

In adults the plaster-of-Paris splint or figure-of-eight is usually satisfactory. It should be maintained for at least four weeks. A residual deformity may be unsightly but rarely interferes with function. Reduction of a gross displacement may occasionally be accomplished by having the patient lie on his back on a narrow table or board with a sandbag between his scapulae and his arms hanging down over the sides of the table. Position can be maintained by any apparatus which will hold the shoulders upward, outward, and backward and permit active function of the extremity.

Occasionally the displacement is so great or the fracture so comminuted that the use of intramedullary wires or some other form of internal fixation may be indicated.

Two methods of treatment are still described in certain textbooks although their use is fortunately becoming less frequent. The Velpeau bandage does not reduce the deformity but tends to increase it. It also immobilizes the entire upper extremity. In other words it is not only useless but harmful. The Sayre dressing may reduce the fracture if sufficiently firmly applied but at the expense of

Injuries to Shoulder Girdle

motion of the arm. If efficiently applied it is almost unbearable for the patient.

Time of Immobilization.—In children three weeks should be adequate. In adults four to six weeks may be necessary. (Active use of the shoulder throughout immobilization is essential.)

Prognosis.—Bony union is the rule with excellent function even in cases with considerable deformity.

Summary.—

Frequent occurrence in children.

Characteristic deformity—forward, downward and inward displacement of shoulder.

Treatment—reduction and appliance holding shoulder back, up and out.

Excellent healing usual.

Good function in spite of deformity.

FRACTURES OF THE SCAPULA

Occurrence.—These infrequent injuries are usually the result of direct violence; for example, a blow from a swinging girder. Indirect violence may be responsible for a certain number, especially of fractures of the scapular neck.

Displacement.—Fractures may occur in the body with or without involvement of the scapular spine; through the neck and glenoid; through the acromion; and, much less commonly, through the coracoid. Fractures through the body may be transverse, oblique or stellate. They show usually little or no displacement of any significance because of the enveloping muscles. If the break involves the neck, the glenoid may be depressed and displaced inward due to the injuring force and the weight of the extremity, with a resulting flattened appearance of the shoulder (Fig. 24). Acromial fragments are apt to be pulled downward by the weight of the arm pulling on the deltoid. The coracoid may show no displacement or may be depressed by the muscles attached to it if the coraco-clavicular ligaments are torn.

Diagnosis.—Tenderness over the body of the scapula, swelling, and pain on motion of the shoulder are suggestive signs. Occasionally bony irregularity can be palpated along the borders of the bone, and in some cases crepitus may be felt during the process of examination.

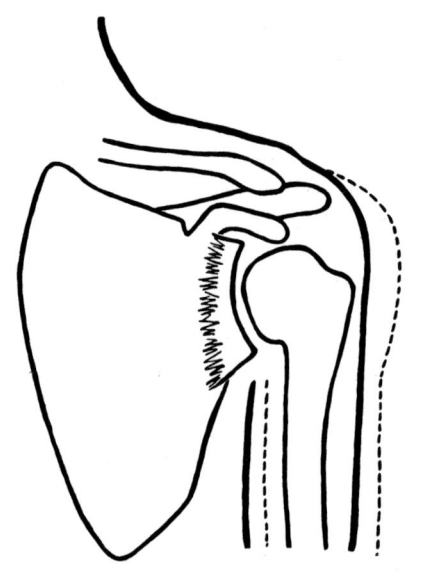

Fig. 24.—Fracture of scapular neck with flattening of the shoulder. Dotted lines indicate the normal contour.

Commolli's sign, a triangular swelling corresponding in size to the scapular body and caused by hemorrhage from the broken bone confined by soft part attachments, is considered by some to be pathognomonic of scapular fracture when it is seen (Fig. 25). It is not present when extensive lacerations of the soft parts permit escape of the blood into the surrounding tissues.

A flattened shoulder with prominent acromion but with the humeral head still in the glenoid is strongly suggestive of fracture of the scapular neck if accompanied by the usual signs of tenderness, swelling and limitation of motion.

Occasionally bony irregularity or actual displacement of the fragment can be felt in acromion and coracoid breaks, but usually local tenderness and swelling are the only leads

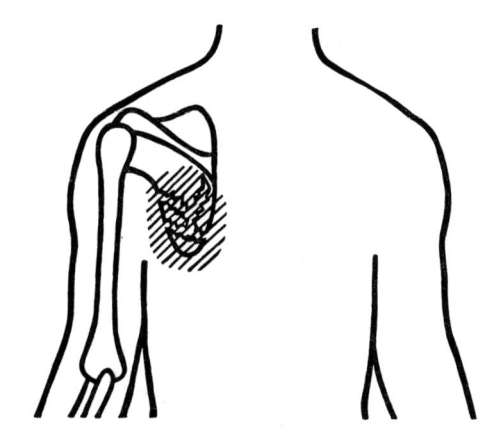

Fig. 25.—Commolli's sign for fracture of the scapula.

and x-ray pictures are necessary to establish the diagnosis.

Pathology.—Because the bone lies as a plate between muscle layers, a fracture is always accompanied by some degree of contusion and laceration of the soft parts. Infiltration of blood into the tissues followed by fibrosis with the resulting diminution of function is characteristic. Nerve and large vessel lesions are uncommon and associated only with extensive injury.

Treatment.—In fractures of the scapular body treatment should be directed toward the soft part pathology. Heat, gentle massage and active motion should be instituted as soon as possible. No form of immobilization is necessary other than a sling to support the arm for a few days. Displacement of the fragments rarely interferes with the functional result.

Fractures of the neck and glenoid should be treated by gentle, continuous traction on the abducted arm. Active motion within pain limits should be encouraged in the traction apparatus.

Acromial and coracoid fractures need only sling support to the arm.

Time of Immobilization.—Sling protection should be used for from two to four weeks.

Prognosis.—Return of function should be complete in two or three months.

Summary.—

Infrequent injuries without characteristic deformity.

Soft part damage of prime importance and treatment directed toward it.

Persistent deformity not incompatible with function.

DISLOCATIONS OF THE CLAVICLE

Acromio-clavicular Joint.—*Occurrence.*—Dislocations at the acromio-clavicular joint are fairly common and are usually caused by a fall or blow on the point of the shoulder depressing the acromion process. Such injuries are frequent in football.

Displacement.—By far the most frequent displacement is an upward shift of the outer end of the clavicle to a varying distance above the acromion. In some cases the clavicle may slip behind the acromion. Downward displacement is extremely rare.

Diagnosis.—The shoulders appear asymmetrical with a prominence of the outer end of the clavicle on the injured side (Fig. 26). This prominence is increased by a downward pull on the arm. Tenderness is localized over the acromio-clavicular joint and there may be moderate swelling and ecchymosis.

X-ray films are of the utmost importance to distinguish between complete (*i.e.*, with torn coraco-clavicular liga-

Injuries to Shoulder Girdle

ments) and incomplete dislocations (with frayed or intact coraco-clavicular ligaments). The x-ray plates should be taken with the patient standing or sitting, his arms hanging by his side, and both shoulders included on the same plate. In complete dislocations there will be an appreciable in-

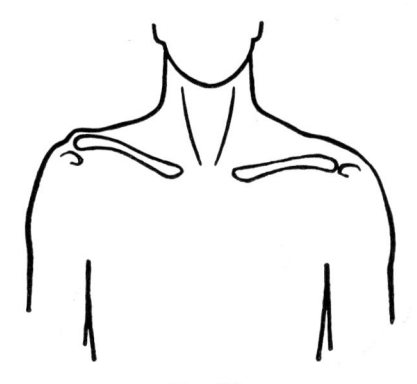

Fig. 26.

crease in the space between the clavicle and the coracoid on the injured side as compared with the uninjured side. In partial dislocations there will be no difference in the coraco-clavicular distance on the two sides though the injured acromio-clavicular joint will appear widened.

Pathology.—In complete dislocations there is always rupture of the coraco-clavicular ligaments as well as of the acromio-clavicular joint capsule. The torn ends are separated and tend to curl under, thereby preventing firm healing. In partial dislocations only slight tearing or stretching of the coraco-clavicular ligaments occurs (Fig. 27, A). Nerve and vessel injuries are rare complications.

Treatment.—In recent complete dislocations operative interference is advised. The outer end of the clavicle can be held in place by two Kirschner wires inserted into it through the acromion. The wires can be left just beneath the skin and removed in eight weeks. Active motion of the

70   Injuries to Shoulder Girdle

extremity should be encouraged from the time of operation (Fig. 27, *D*).

This method because of its simplicity and efficiency has largely supplanted the earlier more elaborate procedures of

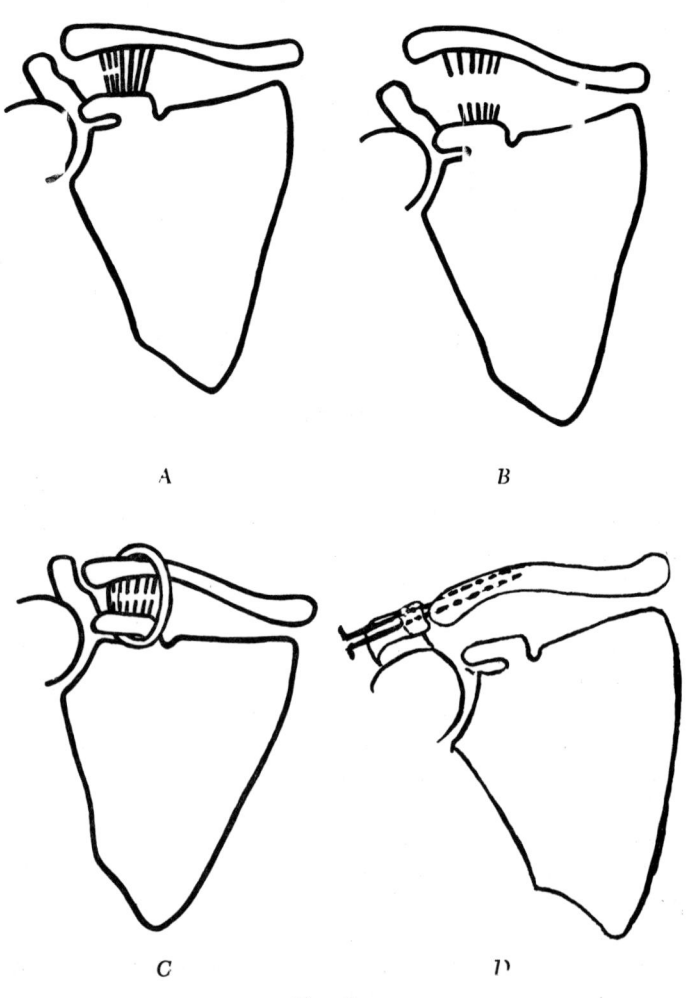

A

B

C

D

Fig. 27.

replacing the torn ligaments by fascia, tendon or silk holding clavicle to coracoid (Fig. 27, *C*).

There are certain surgeons who advocate subperiosteal excision of the outer inch or so of the clavicle in complete dislocations rather than attempting any repair. This is a most satisfactory operation for old dislocations. The functional result is excellent.

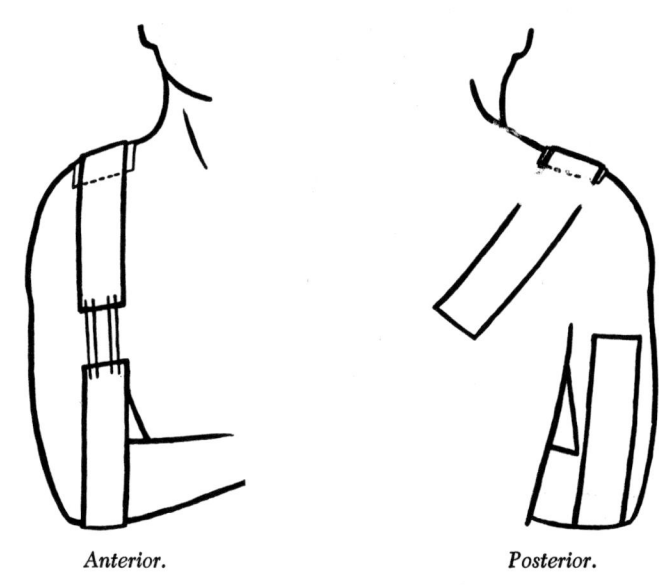

Anterior. *Posterior.*

Fig. 28.—Dressing for incomplete acromio-clavicular dislocation.

Incomplete dislocations may be treated by an adhesive plaster dressing over the shoulder, depressing the clavicle, and under the elbow, lifting the arm (Fig. 28). Careful padding over the olecranon is necessary to avoid pressure sores. Active use of the hand and forearm should be encouraged.

Time of Immobilization.—Some form of dressing should be maintained for from three to four weeks.

Injuries to Shoulder Girdle

Prognosis.—Functional results are almost always excellent in the incomplete and in the repaired complete cases though visible deformity may persist. Pain and weakness of the shoulder may be the result of an unreduced complete dislocation.

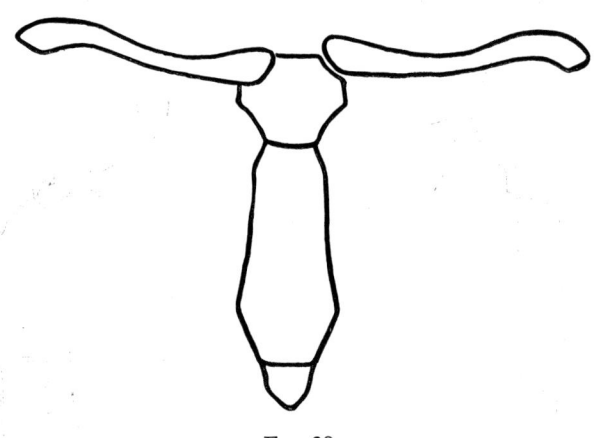

Fig. 29.

Summary.—

Characteristic deformity of prominence of outer end of clavicle.

Incomplete dislocations without complete rupture of coraco-clavicular ligaments treated conservatively.

Complete dislocations with complete rupture of coraco-clavicular ligaments treated operatively.

X-ray picture of both shoulders on same plate essential.

Sterno-clavicular Joint.—*Occurrence.*—These are infrequent injuries and are caused usually by indirect violence. A direct blow may produce a posterior dislocation.

Displacement.—The more usual type is a forward and upward dislocation with the clavicle anterior to and overlying the sternum. It may also be pulled somewhat downward (Fig. 29). Less frequently the sternal end of the clavicle lies posterior to the sternum.

Diagnosis.—A visible and palpable mass at the sterno-clavicular joint is characteristic. Moderate pain and limitation of function also occur but in many cases are not striking. If a posterior dislocation is present the prominence of the sternal border and the posterior position of the clavicle are easily seen and felt.

Pathology.—There is always a stretching or tearing of the sterno-clavicular ligaments and joint capsule. The fibrocartilage usually remains attached to the clavicle. If the displacement is posterior there may be pressure on the trachea, esophagus or vessels.

Treatment.—Reduction of both anterior and posterior dislocations can be accomplished by pressure outward and backward on the shoulders with counterpressure forward between the scapulæ. The position described for reduction of a clavicular fracture may be used. Maintenance of reduction is frequently difficult and can best be attempted by a plaster-of-Paris dressing similar to that described for a clavicular fracture (Fig. 23).

The deformity of a persistent dislocation can be corrected by excision of the inner inch-and-a-half of the clavicle. Operative repair of long-standing dislocations is difficult and not always satisfactory.

Time of Immobilization.—Some form of protection should be maintained for from three to five weeks.

Prognosis.—A moderate prominence is almost inevitable but the function of the extremity is usually complete within a few weeks of the injury.

Summary.—
  Prominence of inner end of clavicle.
  Difficulty of reduction and maintenance of position.
  Deformity rarely a handicap to function.

Chapter 8

Injuries at the Shoulder Joint

FRACTURES OF THE UPPER EXTREMITY OF THE HUMERUS

Anatomical Neck.—*Occurrence.*—This is an uncommon type of fracture and is rarely seen without an associated

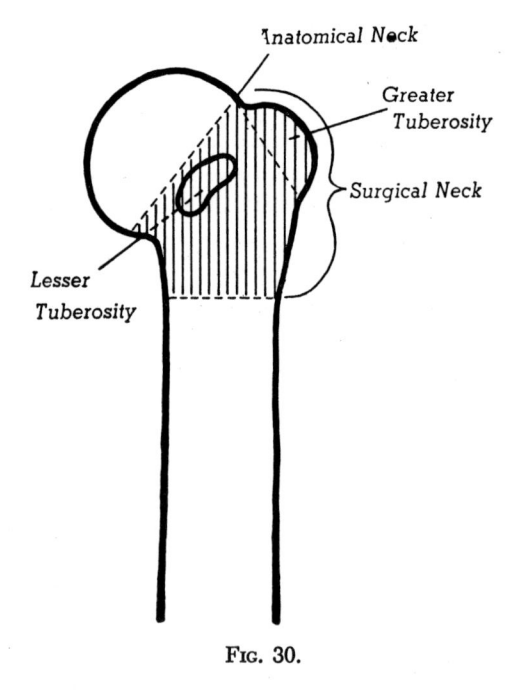

Fig. 30.

dislocation (*q.v.*). High surgical neck fractures are frequently mistaken for it (Fig. 30).

Injuries to the Shoulder Joint

Displacement.—This may be negligible, especially if the fracture is incomplete or impacted.

Diagnosis.—Pain and disability, swelling and tenderness around the shoulder with ecchymosis suggest a fracture of the upper end of the humerus, but x-ray plates are necessary to establish the exact site.

Pathology.—Because of the limited blood supply to the head fragment late changes may take place with resulting flattening of the head or with failure of union.

Treatment.—The earliest possible restoration of motion should be the aim. A sling and body swathe for the first few days with frequent periods of active motion, heat and gentle massage followed by graded exercises can be used in those cases where there is little displacement. When gross displacement has occurred closed reduction, with maintenance of position by traction suspension or some form of ambulatory splint, may be attempted. Operative removal of the head fragment may be necessary.

Time of Immobilization.—These fractures unite fairly rapidly and all protection should be removed in most cases in from three to five weeks.

Prognosis.—This depends largely on the extent of the circulatory damage that has occurred. Abduction is liable to be permanently limited and painful.

Summary.—

Rare injury usually associated with dislocation.

Late deformity possible, due to poor blood supply.

If no displacement, active motion as soon as possible.

Surgical Neck.—*Occurrence.*—These injuries constitute by far the largest number of fractures of the upper end of the humerus. They frequently occur in adults past middle life and are caused in the majority of cases by a fall or blow on the arm.

Displacement.—Impaction may be present with little or no displacement. On the other hand, there may be marked angulation or separation of the fragments. The proximal fragment may be abducted if the greater tuberosity is intact allowing the pull of the supraspinatus to act (Fig. 31). If the greater tuberosity is torn off, however, the head fragment may be actually adducted and internally rotated by the subscapularis. The distal fragment may be pulled inward by the pectoralis and teres major and upward by the

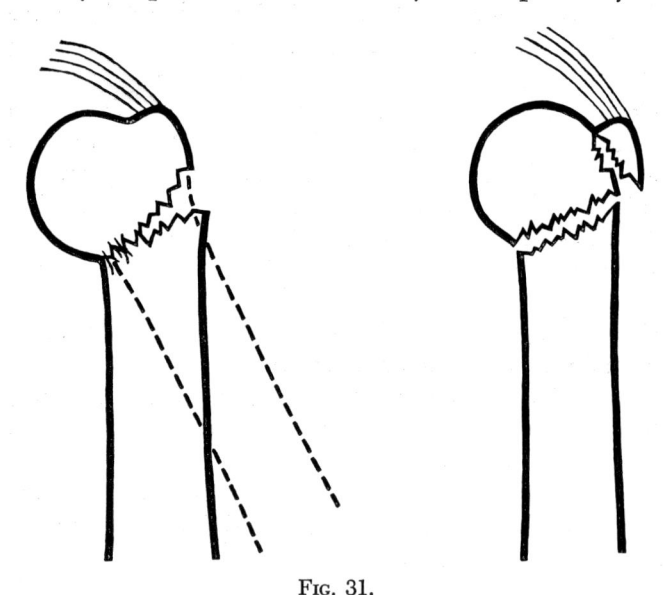

Fig. 31.

biceps and deltoid. The fracturing force, however, undoubtedly plays a large part in the resulting displacement.

Diagnosis.—All elderly patients who complain of pain and disability in the shoulder following a fall should be suspected of having a fracture, especially if there is spreading ecchymosis on the inner side of the arm and on the chest wall twenty-four to forty-eight hours after injury. If there is measurable shortening of the arm, deformity, and no motion of the head when the shaft is gently rotated, the diagnosis of a complete fracture is obvious. X-ray pictures

Injuries to the Shoulder Joint

in two planes if possible, if not, at least in stereo, should always be obtained.

Pathology.—Injury to the brachial plexus and axillary

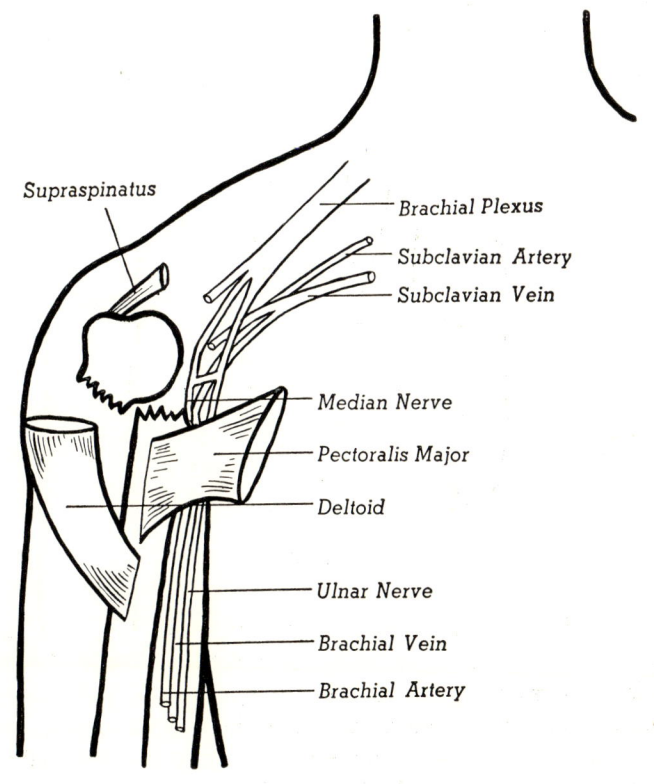

FIG. 32.

vessels from the upper end of the lower fragment may occur if the displacement is great (Fig. 32). Luckily this is a very rare complication. Soft part damage is, however, very frequent with hemorrhage into the surrounding tissues and tearing of bursal walls.

Treatment.—Every effort should be made to regain motion as soon as possible and soft part damage should be combated from the beginning to minimize scarring and fibrosis. The position of abduction should not be used as a routine procedure unless there is a definite indication for it.

When there is impaction, even with considerable malposition of the fragments, treatment by sling and swathe (Fig.

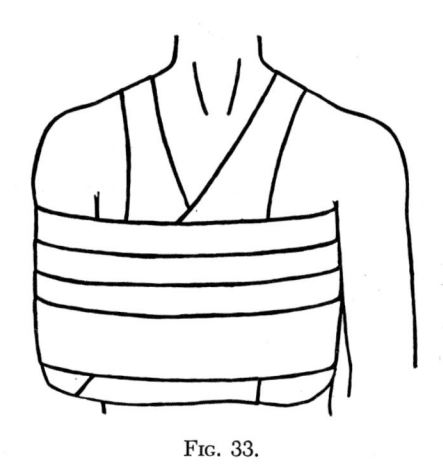

Fig. 33.

33) with pendulum exercises from the first day, heat and gentle massage will give excellent functional results despite bizarre x-ray pictures. If the patient can enter the hospital for suspension and more intensive physical therapy the result may be obtained more rapidly, but the ambulatory treatment under constant supervision is extremely satisfactory.

In cases with displacement, reduction may be accomplished under general anesthetic and held by a sling and swathe if the position is easily maintained or by traction and suspension if the fragments tend to slip. A wire through the lower end of the humerus or through the olecranon is a satisfactory form of traction if skin traction is insufficient to

Injuries to the Shoulder Joint

hold the required position. The position of maintenance depends on the original displacement which must be carefully studied. If the head fragment is adducted or in the mid-position, abduction of the arm will often give a bad angular deformity.

An airplane splint may be used, if abduction is indicated, when bed treatment is for some reason impossible, but these appliances are difficult to fit accurately to the individual. They do not allow the use of extensive physical therapy however, nor motion of the elbow, wrist and fingers. Plaster-of-Paris shoulder spicas are strongly condemned. Their use may give a pretty x-ray picture but will necessitate months of treatment to restore function.

Time of Immobilization.—Impacted fractures need to be protected by a sling and swathe for a week or ten days and by a sling for another two weeks or so. Fractures that have required reduction should be protected for from four to six weeks with active motion within pain limits during that time. Fractures in traction may be placed in sling and swathe when the head and shaft fragments move together.

Prognosis.—Functional return is often surprisingly good in from four to six months in spite of strikingly poor x-ray results.

Summary.—

- Frequent injuries in adults past middle life.
- Deformity dependent on fracturing force and on muscle pull.
- Treatment directed toward functional rather than anatomical restoration.
- Immobilization in abduction indicated only if head fragment is abducted.

Separation of the Epiphysis.—*Occurrence.*—This is a not unusual injury of late childhood and early youth. It is commonly due to a fall on the arm.

Displacement.—This depends largely on the fracturing force. The shaft may be displaced upward and outward or may be tilted on the head fragment to form an angulation opening either medially or laterally. There is almost invariably a fragment of diaphysis remaining on the epiphyseal fragment.

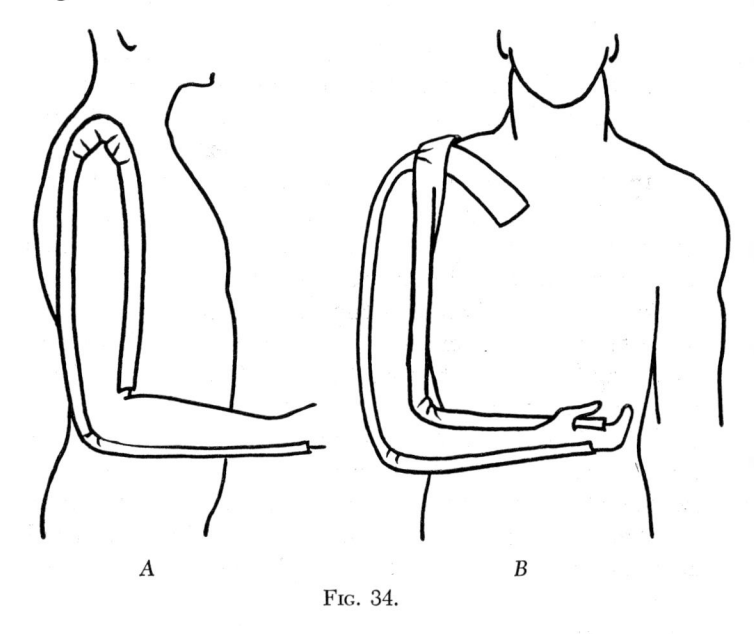

A   B

Fig. 34.

Diagnosis.—The usual signs of fracture at the upper extremity of the humerus in a child or adolescent suggest an epiphyseal injury which may be confirmed by x-ray examination. If the signs are definite but the x-ray evidence is inconclusive or negative, it may be assumed that a fracture has occurred at the epiphyseal line without displacement of the fragments. Subsequent x-ray films may show a faint line of callus.

Pathology.—Frequently soft part damage is not a conspicuous feature though it may be extensive in cases where the displacement of the fragments is great. Nerve injury is uncommon.

Injuries to the Shoulder Joint

Treatment.—Because the injury has taken place through a region of growth, accurate reduction with a minimum of trauma is desirable.

Where no displacement has occurred, *i.e.*, when the diagnosis is clinical and not roentgenographic, a sling and swathe are all that are needed. With a slight displacement easily reduced and held, anterior and posterior molded plaster splints over the shoulder and down the arm or a modified "sugar-tongs" splint will prove satisfactory (Fig. 34).

In cases where gross displacement has occurred, closed reduction under general anesthesia may be necessary. The corrected position can frequently be maintained by a hanging cast or by suspension traction. Open reduction should not be resorted to except in children nearing the end of the growth period, *i.e.* fifteen or sixteen year olds. Damage to the epiphyseal plate at operation may cause more harm in a younger child than the original deformity would if treated conservatively.

Time of Immobilization.—Healing is fairly rapid. Two to three weeks' total protection is usually sufficient in simple cases, four to six weeks for the more severe types.

Prognosis.—As in all cases of epiphyseal injury the prognosis should be guarded as to growth disturbance. Most cases will have a complete return of function in from four to six weeks, but gradual cessation or diminution of growth may occur after several months.

Summary.—

    Reduction advisable by conservative means.

    Operative interference not advised.

    Rapid return of function usual.

    Late growth disturbance possible.

Fractures of the Greater Tuberosity.—*Occurrence.*—This injury is frequently associated with subcoracoid dislocations of the shoulder, but may occur alone. It is caused by muscle pull or by direct violence.

Displacement.—If the fragment is torn completely free from its attachment to the humerus, the muscles attached to it (supraspinatus, infraspinatus and teres minor) will displace it upward and backward. Usually, however, the fragment is only slightly lifted from its bed because its periosteal attachment to the shaft remains intact. If the injury is one of direct violence the tuberosity is depressed rather than pulled off.

Diagnosis.—Acute local tenderness over the outer aspect of the shoulder with pain on attempted abduction and external rotation following an injury to the shoulder is suggestive of fracture. X-ray films of the head of the humerus in internal and external rotation will differentiate between a fracture and a tear of the soft parts.

Pathology.—Hemorrhage into the subdeltoid bursa and the surrounding muscles and tearing of the bursal floor may result from a pulling off of the tuberosity.

Treatment.—Care of the soft part damage should be the chief consideration.

If there is little or no displacement early active motion should be instituted. This is obtained most easily in the first few days by suspension of the extremity so that the weight of the arm is supported. Heat and gentle massage should be prescribed from the beginning. If the fragment is greatly displaced operative replacement with rigid fixation should be considered in order that active motion can be started within a few days. If this is impossible the arm should be held in abduction and external rotation in some form of suspension apparatus or airplane splint.

Time of Immobilization.—In simple cases a sling is usually necessary for about two weeks. If an airplane splint has been used it should be maintained for about three weeks.

Prognosis.—Painful and limited abduction and external rotation may persist for a long time, but in most cases a useful shoulder will be obtained in from three to four months.

Injuries to the Shoulder Joint

Summary.—
Usually associated with dislocation of humeral head.
Fragment displaced up and back by muscles if periosteum is torn.
Soft part pathology important consideration in treatment if fragment is not displaced.

Fractures of the Lesser Tuberosity.—These are rare injuries and are due in most instances to a sudden pull of the subscapularis muscle. The diagnosis is suggested by localized tenderness over the lesser tuberosity and pain on adduction and internal rotation of the arm and is confirmed by x-ray plates. The position of immobilization is that of adduction and internal rotation easily obtained by sling and swathe. Motion within pain limits, heat and massage should be started from the first day.

DISLOCATION OF THE UPPER EXTREMITY OF THE HUMERUS

Anterior or Subcoracoid.—*Occurrence.*—The shoulder is more subject to dislocation than any other joint in the body. The injury occurs preponderantly in young men engaged in strenuous activities but may occur at any age, though rarely seen in childhood. It is caused usually by a fall or blow on the abducted and internally rotated arm.

Displacement.—The head of the humerus is forced out of the antero-inferior part of the capsule and slips forward and upward under the coracoid as the arm drops to the side and the muscles of the shoulder girdle contract.

Diagnosis.—The appearance of a patient with a typical early subcoracoid dislocation is characteristic. The deltoid curve is flattened, the axis of the humerus slants toward the base of the patient's neck instead of toward the acromion process, and there is a prominence instead of a depression visible under the coracoid (Fig. 35). The patient is unable to place the hand of the injured extremity on the opposite shoulder while the elbow is held against the chest (Duga's sign). Gentle palpation reveals the absence of the humeral head in the glenoid and its presence under the coracoid. The head and shaft of the humerus rotate together when the elbow is moved slightly if there is no complicating fracture (Fig. 35). X-ray films, while not essential for the diagnosis, should always be taken to rule out a coëxisting fracture.

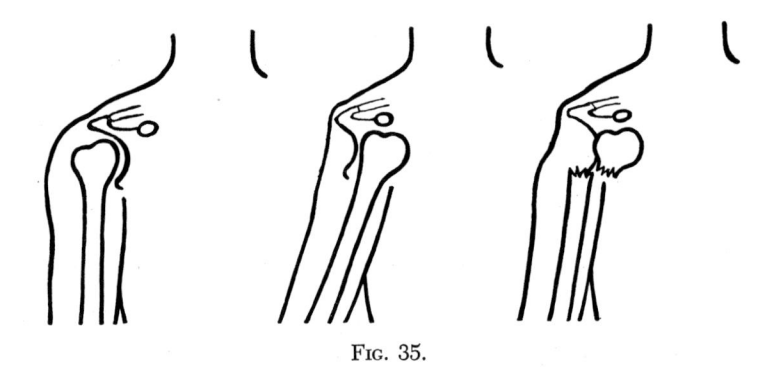

Fig. 35.

Pathology.—The capsule of the shoulder joint is thinnest at the antero-inferior aspect where the subscapularis bursa communicates with the joint. This is the usual site for emergence of the humeral head with tearing of the capsule. The axillary (circumflex) nerve is frequently damaged in the original injury with resulting weakness of the deltoid and anesthesia or hypesthesia over the area of its cutaneous distribution (Fig. 36). The infraclavicular portion of the brachial plexus lies in close proximity to the dislocated head and may be injured in the original trauma, but much more frequently in forcible attempts at reduction.

Treatment.—The essentials of therapy consist of immediate reduction followed by as rapid a restoration to complete function as is consistent with the prevention of a recurrence of the dislocation.

Injuries to the Shoulder Joint 85

Reduction may be done without the use of general anesthesia if the patient is seen soon after the injury or if the dislocation is recurrent. Usually, however, an anesthetic is advisable in order to produce adequate muscular relaxation thereby lessening the force required for the manipulation.

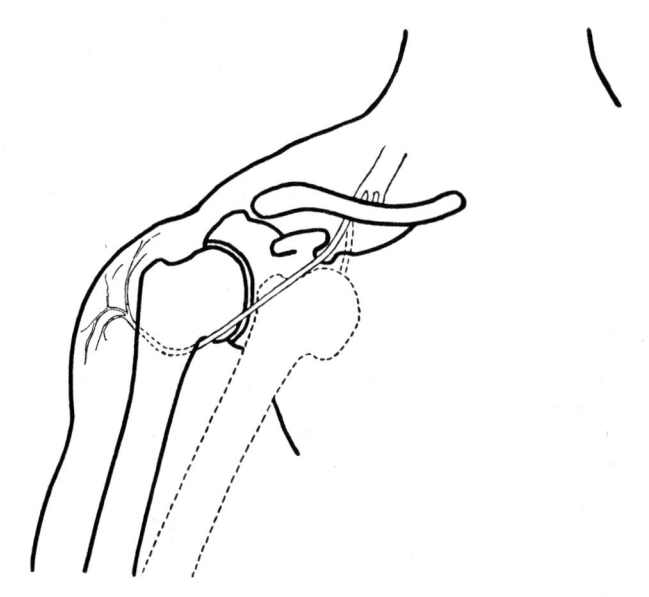

Fig. 36.—Axillary nerve. Showing probability of injury in classical dislocation of shoulder.

All motions to accomplish the reduction should be smooth, slow and steady. Rough and jerky movements are unnecessary and cause damage. Steady traction for five minutes or more in the direction of the axis of the arm will reduce most early dislocations without trouble. Countertraction may be obtained by a swathe tied around the chest over the injured shoulder and fastened to some fixed object or held by an assistant. The "heel-in-the-axilla" method should never be used as there is grave danger of injuring the brachial plexus.

Injuries to the Shoulder Joint

If reduction cannot be accomplished by traction alone the Kocher maneuvers should be tried. They consist of (*a*) external rotation of the arm with the elbow flexed to 90 degrees (Fig. 37); (*b*) adduction, the elbow is moved across the chest (Fig. 38); (*c*) internal rotation, the hand drops to the opposite shoulder (Fig. 39). Steady traction should accompany all the motions and they should be done slowly and smoothly.

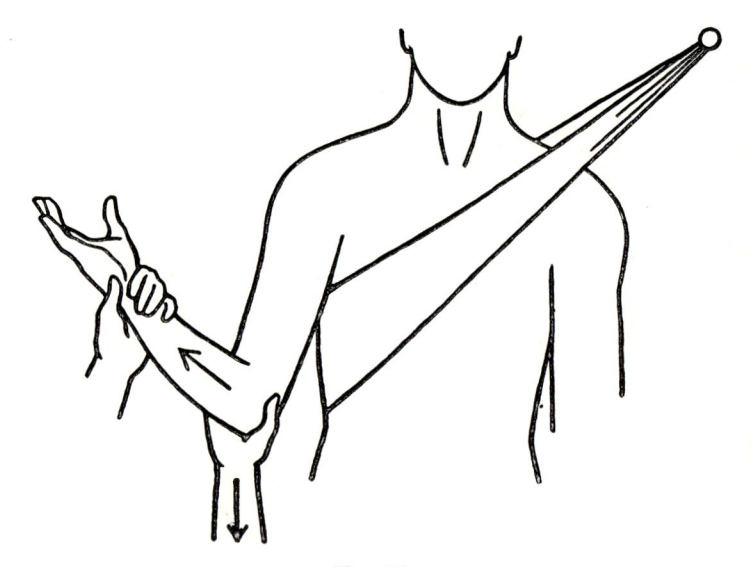

Fig. 37.

If the dislocation has existed for some days, reduction may be impossible by the above methods without the use of undue force. In such cases skin traction of 10 to 15 pounds applied over a period of hours is valuable to relax the muscles and slowly stretch the soft parts.

In the early cases after reduction a sling and swathe should be used for two or three days followed by a sling for another week or ten days. Heat, massage and active motion

Injuries to the Shoulder Joint 87

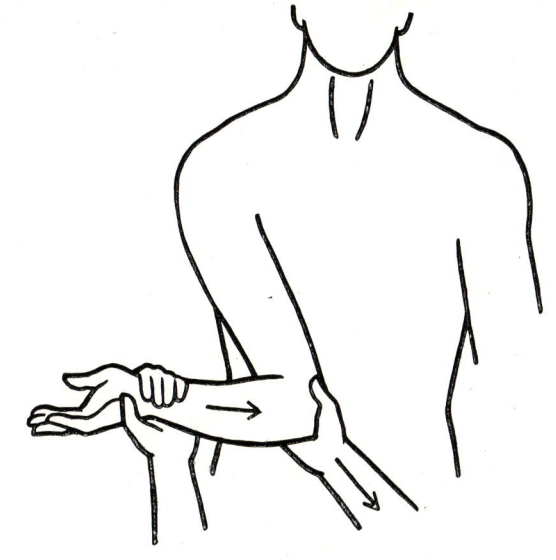

Fig. 38.

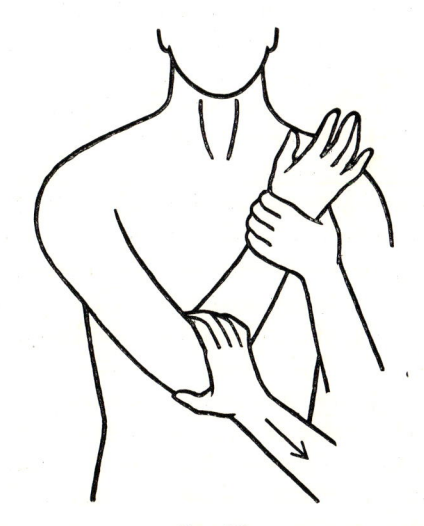

Fig. 39.

within pain limits should be instituted from the beginning. The patient should be warned against abduction beyond 90 degrees for from four to six weeks because of the danger of recurrence. If there is evidence of axillary nerve damage or much soft part trauma the patient should be admitted to a hospital for suspension of the arm at 70 degrees' abduction to allow intensive physical therapy and to relax the strain on the deltoid.

Time of Immobilization.—Sling protection for two or three weeks is usually adequate with abduction limited for four or six weeks.

Prognosis.—Full functional return in from six to eight weeks is the usual result in early cases. Recurrences are not infrequent, however, and the patient should be warned against them.

Recurrent dislocations are best treated for permanent cure by operative means.

Summary.—
- Most frequent of all dislocations.
- Deformity striking; flattening of shoulder, bulge under coracoid, axis of arm through base of neck.
- Axillary nerve injury common.
- Reduction by steady traction usually easy.
- Sling and swathe for a few days.
- Recurrence not uncommon.

Inferior or Subglenoid.—In these cases the head of the humerus remains where it has emerged from the joint and does not slip up under the coracoid. The arm appears longer than the other side but in all other respects appearance and treatment are similar to those of the subcoracoid type.

Posterior.—These dislocations are rare but should never be missed if a practice is made of looking at all injured shoulders from the side as well as from front and back. The deformity is then obvious, as the bulge formed by the humeral head is seen well behind the acromion. Reduction can be accomplished by steady traction on the arm but may

Injuries to the Shoulder Joint

be difficult to maintain if there is an associated fracture of the glenoid lip.

Complications of Shoulder Dislocations.—*Fracture of the Greater Tuberosity.*—This is of frequent occurrence and offers no contraindication to the immediate reduction of the dislocation. Usually the fragment slips back into place without difficulty (Fig. 40). Suspension of the arm in 70 degrees' abduction for several days with intensive physical therapy will materially shorten the period of convalescence.

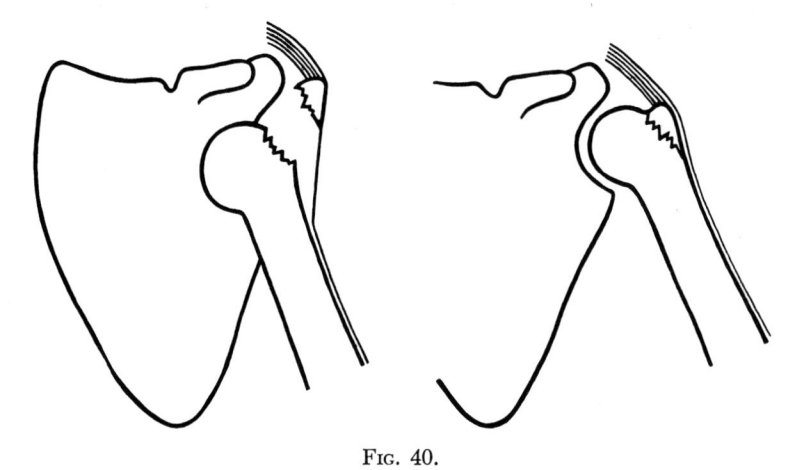

Fig. 40.

Fracture of the Glenoid.—Occasionally a fragment is broken from the rim of the glenoid and may make a reduction impossible to maintain without operative interference.

Fracture of the Anatomical or of the Surgical Neck.—These cases form one of the most difficult problems in all fracture surgery. The diagnosis is suggested by the signs of a subcoracoid dislocation modified by shortening of the arm, by a failure of the head to rotate with the shaft, and occasionally by crepitus. X-ray pictures confirm the diagnosis. Occasionally manipulative reduction can be accomplished in an early case if great care is used to prevent further damage.

Frequently, however, operation is necessary. If there is sufficient soft part attachment to the head fragment to provide adequate blood supply it should be replaced if possible. If the fracture is high, *i.e.*, through the anatomical neck, it is wiser to remove the fragment because of the danger of late changes in the head with increasing disability.

Displacement of the Long Head of the Biceps.—Rarely the long head of the biceps is torn out of the bicipital groove and becomes displaced behind the humeral head. Reduction can be effected but cannot be maintained, as any action of the biceps flips the head out of the joint. Operative interference is necessary in such cases.

Chapter 9

Fractures of the Shaft of the Humerus

Occurrence.—These injuries occur usually in active adult life. They are caused for the most part by severe violence, either direct or indirect. Rarely a fracture may be caused by muscle action, especially in the upper third when the bone is weakened by a solitary cyst.

Displacement.—Occasionally, particularly in children, there may be no displacement. Usually, however, if the fracture is complete the fragments tend to override because of the strength of the muscle pull. If the fracture line is above the deltoid insertion there is a tendency for the lower fragment to be displaced outward. For the most part the displacement is determined by the fracturing force. Comminution is a frequent finding.

Diagnosis.—If there is displacement the diagnosis can be made at a glance for the deformity is obvious. In cases with no deformity x-ray films are essential to differentiate between a fracture and a soft part injury.

Pathology.—The radial (musculospiral) nerve winds around the shaft of the humerus close to the bone between the internal and external heads of the triceps. In fractures of the middle third of the shaft the nerve is frequently injured at the time of the original trauma (Fig. 41), during manipulative reduction, or later by pressure of the callus. Interposition of soft parts between the bone ends is a not infrequent finding.

Delayed and non-union are relatively frequent in fractures of the humeral shaft and are unfortunate complications.

Fractures of Shaft of the Humerus

Treatment.—In cases where there is no displacement, particularly in fractured humeral shafts in children, anterior and posterior molded splints or sugar tongs splints (see Fig. 34) are adequate. Adduction of the elbow with angulation at the fracture site may be prevented by the use of a triangular axillary pad. These splints should be worn for six weeks.

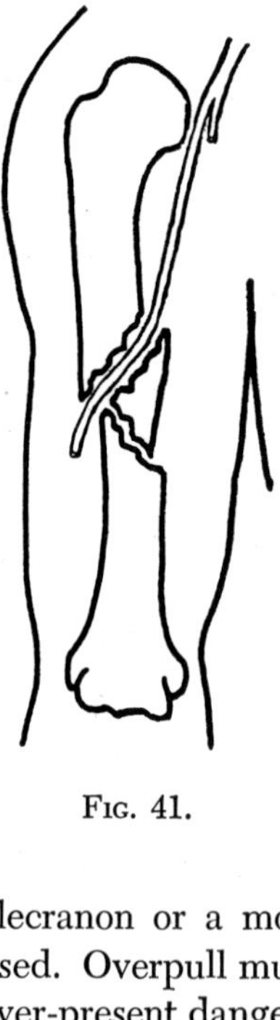

Where displacement has occurred in children and in adults the hanging plaster casing (Fig. 42) is satisfactory in many cases. The plaster should exert a continuous traction which means that the patient should sleep in a semi-sitting position to allow the extremity to hang. The plaster must be suspended from the wrist and the usual sling discarded. Movements of fingers and shoulder should be encouraged to prevent stiffness.

If there is gross displacement with comminution, and if plaster is not applicable due to the presence of a wound, wire traction through the olecranon or a modified form of Russell traction may be used. Overpull must be guarded against as non-union is an ever-present danger.

If there is radial nerve damage and/or evidence of interposition of soft parts, operative interference with rigid internal fixation, if possible, is indicated. Under suitable conditions operation with internal fixation may be chosen as the method of choice in any case with gross displacement.

Time of Immobilization.—Six to eight weeks if internal fixation is not used.

Prognosis.—Full use of the extremity is usually attained

Fig. 41.

Fractures of Shaft of the Humerus

in from three to four months if there has been no nerve lesion and if non-union does not supervene.

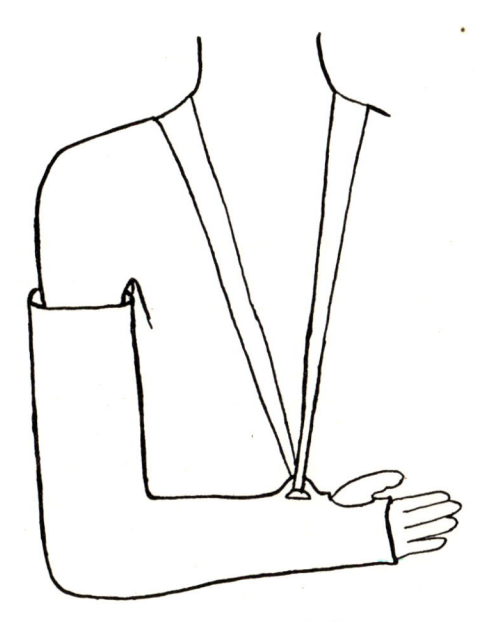

Fig. 42.—"Hanging" plaster.

Summary.—
  Injuries caused by considerable violence.
  Radial nerve damage not uncommon in fractures at the mid-third of the shaft.
  Hanging plaster frequently satisfactory, skeletal traction or operation with internal fixation may be necessary.
  Delayed or non-union not infrequent.

Chapter 10

Injuries at the Elbow Joint

FRACTURES OF THE LOWER EXTREMITY OF THE HUMERUS

Supracondylar or Dicondylar Fractures.—*Occurrence.*—These are common accidents of childhood. They are caused by a fall on the hand or forearm, very rarely by a fall or blow on the back of the elbow.

Displacement.—The lower end of the humerus curves forward so that from a lateral view a line through the capitellum forms an angle with the axis of the shaft. The direction of the fracturing force is usually such that the distal fragment is displaced backward. There may be only angulation, *i.e.*, the capitellum may lie in line with the axis of the shaft (Fig. 43), or there may be complete separation with overriding (Fig. 44). Lateral or medial shift of the distal fragment may occur and frequently there is a rotary displacement of the lower end of the humerus on the shaft.

Anterior displacement is a rare occurrence and is due to a force directed from behind.

Diagnosis.—There are certain landmarks around the elbow joint which are important aids in diagnosis. The two epicondyles can be easily palpated even when there is considerable swelling. Normally they lie in line with the shaft of the humerus (Fig. 45). The olecranon process can also be palpated. With the elbow flexed the tip of the olecranon lies equidistant between the two epicondyles and the three points form an isosceles triangle (Figs. 46 and 47). With the elbow extended the tip of the olecranon lies on the line joining the epicondyles (Figs. 48 and 49). When the elbow is extended and the forearm supinated the forearm normally

Injuries to the Elbow Joint 95

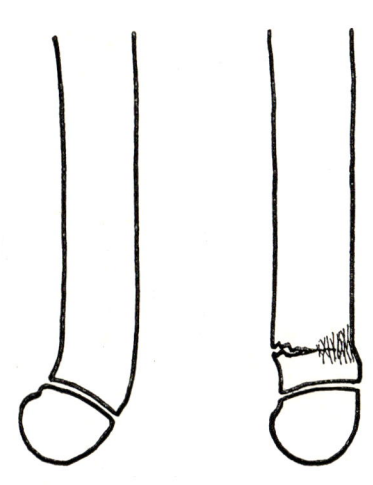

Fig. 43.

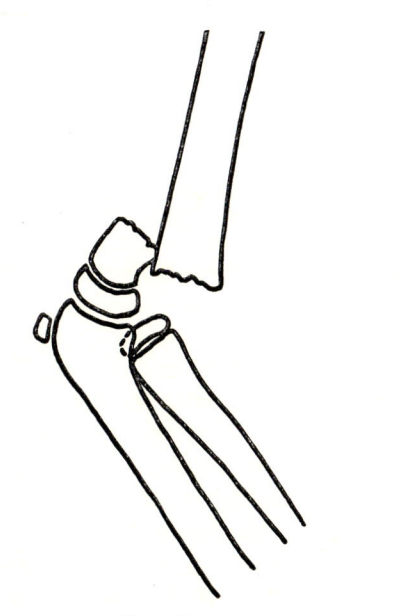

Fig. 44.

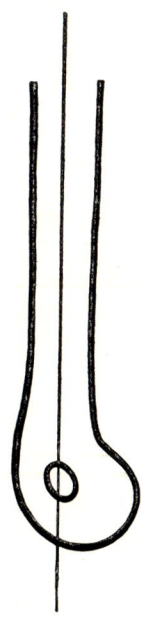

Fig. 45.

swings slightly outward, so that its axis forms an angle with a continuation of the axis of the arm of from 5 to 20 degrees, the "carrying angle." When the elbow is completely flexed and the forearm supinated the hand drops to the acromion process.

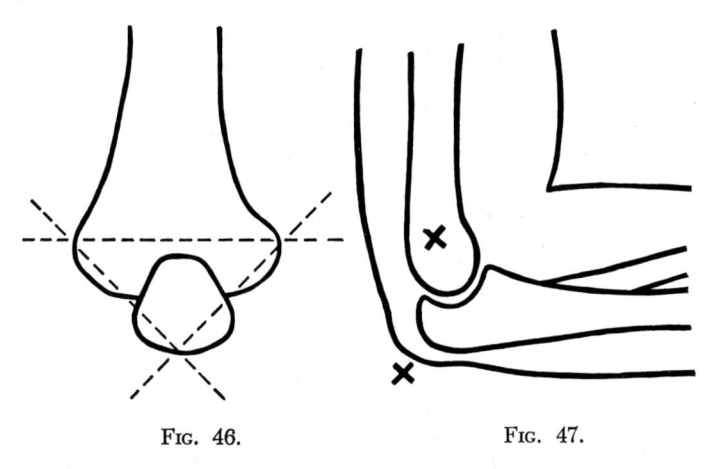

FIG. 46.   FIG. 47.

In a supracondylar fracture with gross displacement, backward displacement of the elbow is visible. On palpation it is found that the relationship between the epicondyles and the olecranon is normal but that the epicondyles lie posterior to the axis of the humerus (Fig. 50). There may be measurable shortening of the arm.

If there is little or no displacement, linear tenderness across the lower end of the humerus, both anteriorly and posteriorly, and indirect tenderness, elicited by gentle pressure on the olecranon with the elbow flexed, suggest the diagnosis. X-ray plates are always necessary.

Pathology.—Because of the usual character of the displacement the brachial artery may be occluded either by direct pressure against the distal end of the proximal fragment or by local spasm. Hemorrhage and edema beneath the lacertus fibrosus (bicipital fascia) may hinder venous

Injuries to the Elbow Joint 97

and lymphatic drainage. Volkmann's ischemic paralysis, the result of prolonged circulatory embarrassment, is one of the most tragic accidents in the surgery of trauma. Acute flexion of the elbow constricting the artery or too tight

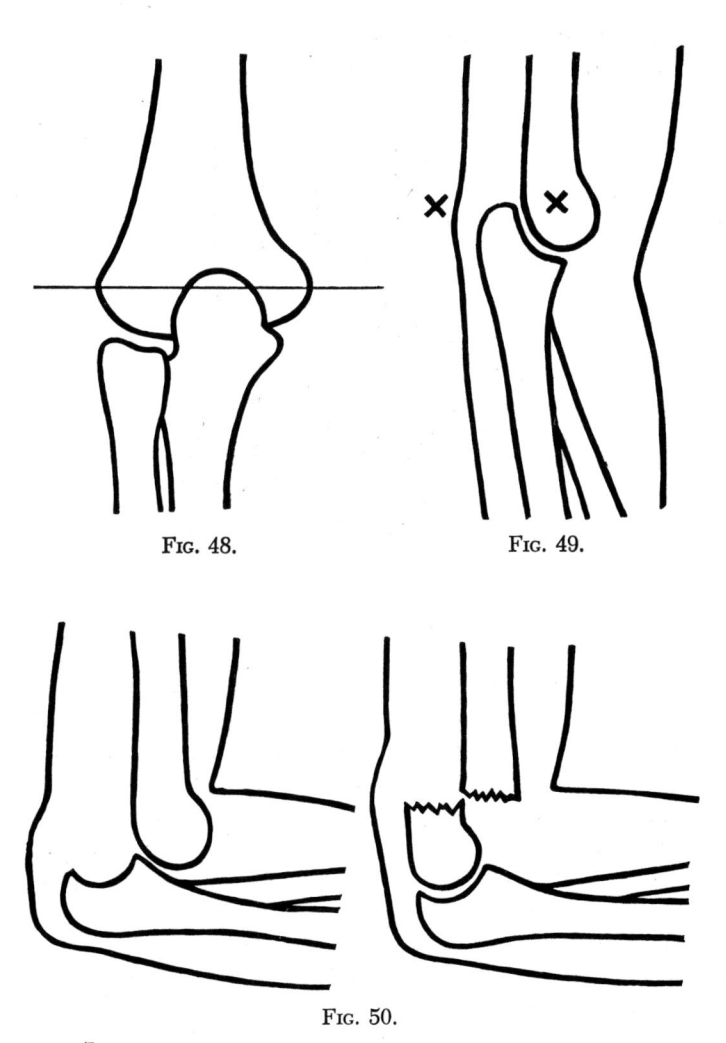

FIG. 48.   FIG. 49.

FIG. 50.

bandages may be contributory factors but the primary cause is usually arterial spasm. Nerve damage in supracondylar fractures may occur but less frequently than circulatory damage.

Treatment.—Early accurate reduction is essential in these cases. As the majority of patients are children, the functional return is satisfactory if the deformity is corrected.

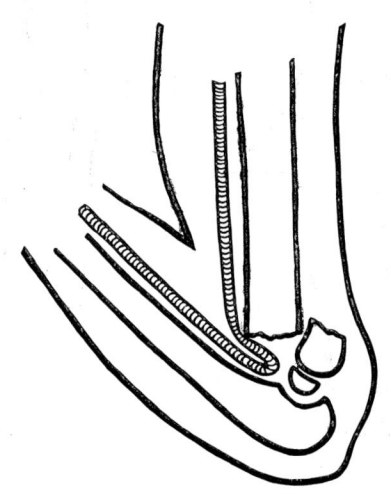

Fig. 51.—Possible effect of flexion on the brachial artery.

Palpation of the radial pulse and examination of the fingers for color, temperature, sensation and motion should always be part of the original examination. If the radial pulse is not palpable or is very weak, speed of reduction is even more important than in the uncomplicated case.

In many cases reduction by manipulation under an anesthetic can be done satisfactorily. Traction on the distal fragment must be maintained throughout the maneuver to release the impinging bone ends. Care must be taken to correct rotation of the fragment as well as posterior and lateral or medial displacements. Flexion of the elbow is a

Injuries to the Elbow Joint

position of maintenance, not of reduction (Fig. 51), and should not be done until the fragments are in line. When a satisfactory position has been obtained the elbow should be flexed with the radial pulse under palpation during the procedure. Should the pulse grow weak or disappear, the flexion should be reduced until the pulse is again maximum. The position can be held by a posterior molded splint from shoulder to knuckles. Circular plaster should never be used. Figure-of-eight adhesive strips are unsatisfactory as swelling occurs between the strips and internal rotation of the lower fragment may take place when the forearm swings across the chest. The forearm should be in supination or pronation, whichever holds the position better. Usually supination is satisfactory. Every effort should be made to avoid any constricting plaster or bandage in the antecubital fossa.

Following reduction and splinting, the arm should be elevated, and the patient kept under close observation for at least twenty-four hours. Pulse, color and temperature of the fingers should be frequently observed and the bandage cut down at the slightest suggestion of diminished circulation. Volkmann's paralysis can occur in a few hours.

If a satisfactory position has been obtained and held, while a good radial pulse persists, the splint should be left in place for about three weeks and then replaced by a sling for another two or three weeks with active flexion encouraged during that period. Physical therapy is definitely contraindicated.

If reduction cannot be obtained by manipulation or if it cannot be maintained at the degree of flexion necessary to get the maximal radial pulse, traction by means of a Kirschner wire through the base of the olecranon is extremely satisfactory. The arm should be suspended over the bed so that circulatory drainage is obtained (Fig. 52). Anatomical reposition can be achieved in a few hours by adjusting the line of pull. In these cases traction should be continued for ten days to two weeks and then replaced by a posterior molded splint holding the elbow in flexion of less than 90°. A sling can be substituted for the splint in about two weeks.

If the radial pulse is not palpable on the first examination and does not return within one-half hour of traction and suspension, operative slitting of the fascia of elbow and fore-

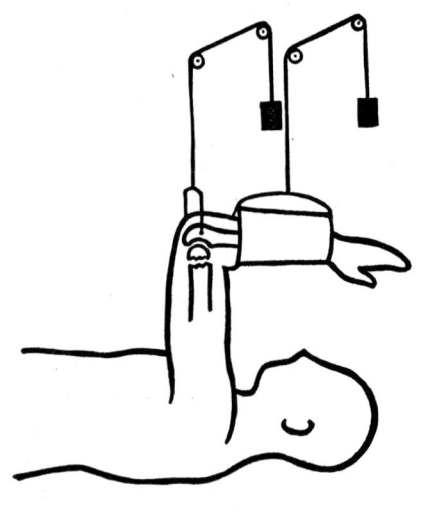

Fig. 52.

arm should be considered. Stellate ganglion blocks may obviate the need for operation. There is no excuse for waiting "until the swelling goes down," for the swelling is largely due to the deformity. The quickest way to reduce the swelling is to reduce the fracture.

The results of open reductions of supracondylar fractures in children are most disappointing, and therefore operative interference for the purpose of correcting poor position is not advised.

Complete functional return is likely to be slow and should not be rushed by any forceful means. Manipulations to

Injuries to the Elbow Joint

increase elbow motion are dangerous and unnecessary. Use of the extremity in normal activities is usually all that is needed to restore full range of motion. If the child is timid and continues to protect the injured elbow, confinement of the uninjured arm in a sling beneath the shirt is a simple and valuable expedient.

Time of Immobilization.—Undisplaced fractures should be splinted from two to three weeks followed by a sling for another couple of weeks. More complicated cases should have splint protection from three to four weeks.

Prognosis.—If a satisfactory reduction is obtained the result should be good both anatomically and functionally in from four to six months. Occasionally growth disturbances and inaccurate reduction result in unsightly elbows, most frequently in a reversed carrying angle or "gun stock" deformity.

Complications of Supracondylar Fractures.—Volkmann's ischemic paralysis, caused by interference with the circulation by pressure either from within or from without, may occur within a few hours after injury and cause permanent damage to forearm and hand. Massive replacement of muscle fibers by fibrous tissue makes late correction difficult and in some cases impossible. This complication should always be watched for and prevented.

Myositis ossificans, the formation of bone in muscle, may occur in the fibers of the brachialis. Forced passive motions and deep massage seem to be favorable to its formation. The bony mass increases in size for from six to nine months after onset, remains stationary about three months, and then regresses. Normal use of the extremity is the only treatment. Operative removal should never be attempted during the period of growth of the mass for recurrence is almost inevitable. Frequently the osseous tissue will completely disappear spontaneously. If not, it can be removed when it has reached its minimum size.

Summary.—
 A common injury of childhood.
 Backward and rotary displacement of distal fragment usual.
 Immediate accurate reduction and immobilization in flexion satisfactory in most cases.
 Wire traction through the upper extremity of ulna valuable in difficult cases.
 Circulatory damage a danger which must be anticipated and prevented.
 Anatomical restoration important to prevent unsightly deformity.

T or Y Fractures.—*Occurrence.—*These fractures are most frequently found in adults and are caused by a blow or fall on the flexed elbow or by a fall on the hand.

*Displacement.—*The condyles are often spread apart with the ulna jammed up between them or the upper humeral fragment pushed down.

*Diagnosis.—*In severe cases broadening of the lower end of the humerus is apparent. There may be a changed relationship between the epicondyles and the olecranon. Tenderness on lateral pressure over the epicondyles is present and occasionally the condyles can be felt to move toward each other on such pressure. Shortening of the arm may be measurable. Roentgenographs are essential for details of the injury.

*Pathology.—*As in most elbow injuries there is marked swelling. Rarely one or more of the nerves may be injured in the original trauma.

*Treatment.—*In adults functional return is more important than anatomical restoration. A perfectly reduced fracture immobilized over a period of weeks may result in a stiff elbow. Therefore, while closed reduction and immobilization may be possible, some form of treatment to allow early return of motion is preferable. Traction and suspension by Dunlop's method with skin traction (Fig. 53), by a Mag-

Injuries to the Elbow Joint

nuson felt, or by a Kirschner wire through the olecranon are valuable methods in certain cases.

Traction should be maintained for from three to five weeks and then the patient allowed up with the elbow protected by a posterior molded splint which should be removed daily for active exercise. All protection should be off

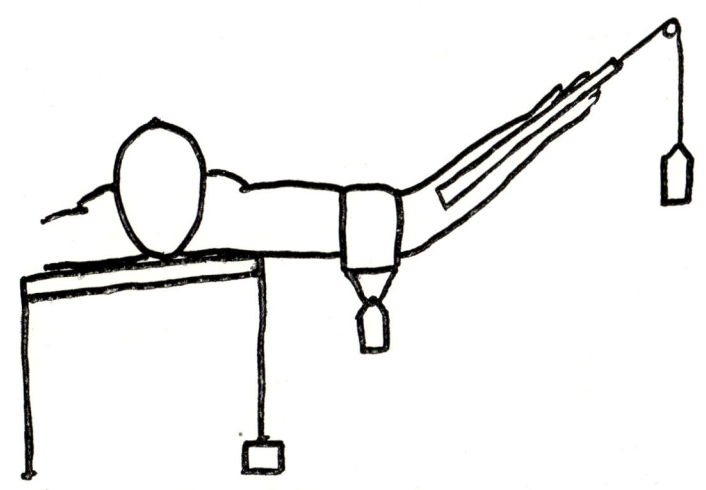

FIG. 53.—Dunlop's method of elbow traction.

in eight weeks. In other cases operative reduction with some form of internal fixation by means of nails, screws or pegs may be necessary, though frequently mechanically difficult because of the shape of the fragments. Early active motion must be stressed.

Time of Immobilization.—This varies with the extent of the injury but in most instances should be solid enough in from six to eight weeks to allow the patient to go without any protection.

Prognosis.—These are serious injuries and seldom result in a perfect extremity. Careful treatment should give a useful arm but almost always extension remains limited.

Summary.—
- Serious injuries in adults.
- Wire traction through olecranon useful.
- Operative fixation necessary in certain cases.
- Function more important than anatomical restoration.
- Prolonged immobilization to be avoided because of danger of a stiff joint.

Fractures of the Condyles.—EXTERNAL CONDYLE.—*Occurrence.*—This is not an infrequent accident, usually of childhood. It is caused by a force directed upward against the outer side of the articular surface of the humerus or by a hyperadduction of the forearm.

Displacement.—The fracture line runs upward from the joint surface just medial to the capitellum, including the capitellar epiphysis, and slants outward to the external supracondylar ridge.

Any degree of separation may occur, from a slight crack to a complete rotation of 180 degrees. The pull of the extensor muscles of the forearm tends to pivot the fragment laterally, so that in extreme cases the fracture surface may face outward (Fig. 54).

Diagnosis.—Tenderness and swelling localized to the outer side of the elbow, with or without palpable displacement of the lateral condyle, suggest this injury. X-ray examination is necessary to determine the amount of displacement.

Pathology.—The extensor group of muscles attaches to the external supracondylar ridge and some part of the attachment is frequently torn off with the fragment. Nerve injuries are rare.

Treatment.—Accurate replacement of the fragment is necessary to prevent the deformity of an increased carrying angle, which may result years later in ulnar nerve damage. Where the displacement is negligible a posterior molded splint holding the elbow in moderate flexion, and maintained for from two to three weeks, is all that is required.

Injuries to the Elbow Joint

Where there is marked separation and rotation of the fragment immediate reduction by manipulation under an anesthetic may be tried, but is rarely successful. Open operation with replacement and fixation of the fragment is usually necessary. Removal of the fragment should be done only in late cases where the chance of obtaining an accurate reposition is negligible.

Time of Immobilization.—A splint for about three weeks is usually advisable, followed by a sling for another week.

Prognosis.—Functional return is good in three to four months as a rule, but a prominence of the external condyle to greater or lesser degree is a frequent result. If an increased carrying angle results due to an upward slipping of the condyle, there may be late ulnar nerve symptoms due to stretching.

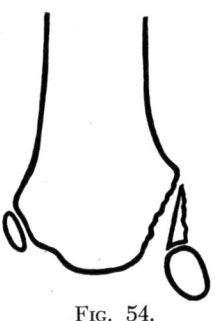

FIG. 54.

Summary.—

Rotary displacement due to muscle pull.

Operative fixation frequently necessary.

Ulnar nerve symptoms a possible late complication.

INTERNAL CONDYLE.—These are rare injuries, usually occurring in adults and requiring operative replacement and fixation if the fragment is markedly displaced.

INTERNAL EPICONDYLE.—*Occurrence.*—A common injury in childhood, this fracture is caused by a forcible abduction of the forearm, tearing off the fragment (usually the epiphysis) by muscle pull. It may be associated with dislocation at the elbow joint.

Displacement.—The fragment is pulled downward by the flexor muscles. Rarely, usually associated with dislocation of the forearm bones, the fragment is pulled into the joint and lies between ulna and trochlea (Fig. 55).

Diagnosis.—Localized tenderness and swelling over the medial aspect of the elbow with prominence of the internal

Injuries to the Elbow Joint

epicondyle are suggestive. X-ray films are essential. The characteristic kidney bean or semi-oval shape of the epicondyle distinguishes it from the semicircular or pie-shaped fragments of the radial head for which it might be mistaken (Fig. 55).

Pathology.—There may be very little swelling with this injury unless there has been considerable soft part damage. Occasionally the ulnar nerve is injured.

Treatment.—If there is

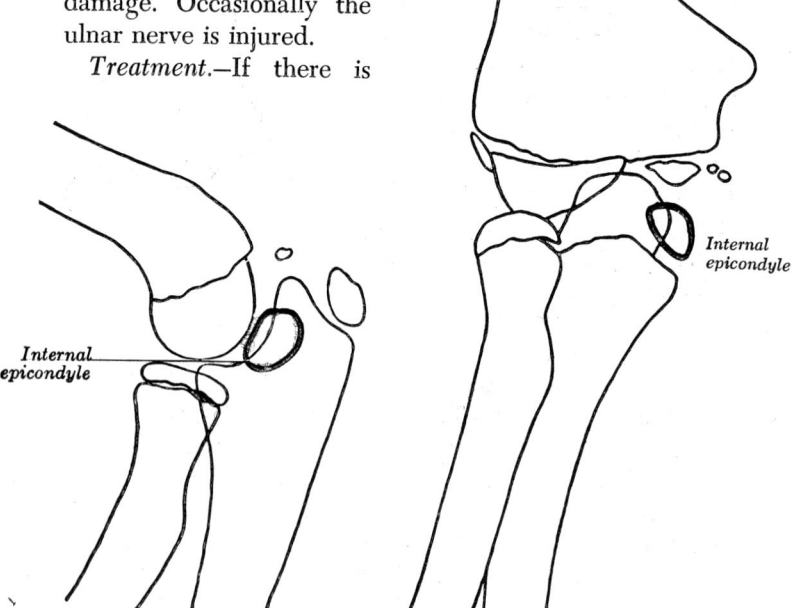

Fig. 55.

little or no displacement no splint is necessary, but the use of a sling for four or five days is advised. If there is gross separation of the epicondyle an attempt can be made to manipulate it up into position. A posterior splint should then be applied, holding the elbow at a little less than 90

Injuries to the Elbow Joint

degrees and the forearm pronated. The splint should be maintained for about a week and followed by a sling and active exercises.

If the fragment lies in the joint early operation is indicated. The epiphysis should usually not be removed but sutured into place. Some advocate removal of the bone fragment with suture of the soft tissues. Treatment should be continued as in the uncomplicated cases.

Time of Immobilization.—A splint should be maintained for about a week, followed by a sling and active exercises.

Prognosis.—Return of function is usually excellent even with a fibrous union of the fragments. Full extension may be slow in returning, as is frequently the case in all elbow injuries.

Summary.—

Displacement downward due to muscle pull, occasionally in the joint after dislocation of both bones.

Closed reduction in simple cases.

Operative reduction when in the joint.

Ulnar nerve injury a possible complication.

Separation of the Epiphysis Without Displacement.—*Occurrence.*—These injuries are quite common and are frequently diagnosed as sprains or bruises. They are usually due to a fall on the extended hand.

Diagnosis.—Tenderness at the lower end of the humerus which extends across the bone both anteriorly and posteriorly, and is accompanied by swelling, suggests a possible fracture. With definite signs of fracture but a negative x-ray plate, the possibility of a break across the epiphyseal cartilage must be considered.

Pathology.—There is always moderate swelling but gross circulatory damage does not occur. Nerve injuries also are not found. X-ray films taken ten days to two weeks after the injury frequently show a faint line of callus running up the humeral shaft.

Treatment.—These cases should be treated like supracondylar fractures without displacement, *i.e.*, with a posterior molded splint for two weeks. They may be slow in regaining complete extension, but attempts to hurry the return of function by physical therapy should not be made.

Time of Immobilization.—Splint protection is necessary for about two weeks.

Prognosis.—Full functional return is the rule but may be slower than the parents anticipate. Rarely growth disturbances may occur.

Summary.—

Frequent injuries showing signs and symptoms of fracture but no x-ray evidence.

Splint protection for two weeks.

Functional return complete but growth disturbance a possibility.

FRACTURES OF THE UPPER EXTREMITY OF THE RADIUS

Fractures of the Radial Head.—*Occurrence.*—These injuries are fairly frequent and are likely to be overlooked. They are caused by a fall on the hand or forearm and may be associated with a dislocation at the elbow.

Displacement.—The fragments may be completely separated from the head or merely depressed. The position depends on the fracturing force. Frequently the fracture is represented by a crack through the articular surface with no displacement (Fig. 56).

Diagnosis.—The presence of a distended joint capsule associated with limitation of motion, especially pronation and supination, and tenderness over the radial head, following a fall, suggests a fracture. A characteristic symptom is that of gradually increasing pain two or three hours after the injury, caused by the increasing pressure in the joint from the hemarthrosis. X-ray pictures are not always con-

Injuries to the Elbow Joint

clusive as they may not show a small crack. The diagnosis should be made on clinical evidence.

Pathology.—If there is no displacement, blood in the joint is the principal evidence of damage. If the fragment is displaced anteriorly, especially if the capsule is torn, there is usually considerable injury to the soft parts in the front of the elbow. In such cases excessive bone production or overgrowth is a danger. Because of the tearing of the capsule the blood escapes into the tissues and there will not be a hemarthrosis. Rarely there is damage to the radial nerve.

Treatment.—1. *Fractures Without Displacement.*—If there is sufficient fluid in the joint to cause limitation of motion and pain, the joint should be aspirated. A posterior molded splint for the first two or three days tends to prevent further bleeding into the joint and provides rest and protection. After that a sling for a week or ten days is all that is needed for immobilization. Active motion within pain limits should be started after twenty-four hours.

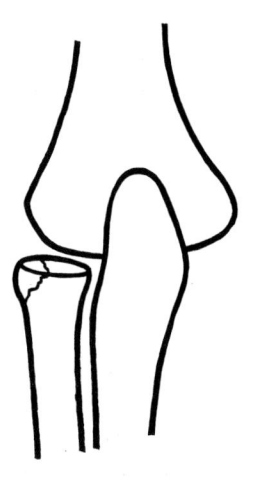

Fig. 56.

2. *Fractures With Displacement.*—If there is gross displacement of a considerable portion of the head the best procedure is operative removal, usually of the entire head. There are some who advocate removing the fragment only, when it is small. Closed reduction of the fracture is almost invariably impossible in adults. Operation should be performed within the first few days following injury or several months later, not in the active bone-forming period. If there is anterior displacement of the fragments with injury to the soft parts in the antecubital fossa, the sooner the operation can be done the less danger there is of bony

overgrowth. Following operation active motion should be started as soon as possible.

Time of Immobilization.—A splint is necessary for only two or three days in most cases. A sling may be used for from one to two weeks.

Prognosis.—Return of full extension of the elbow may be delayed for months even in those cases where there is no displacement of the fragment. However, full return of motion may be expected in from six months to a year in the usual uncomplicated fracture. In operative cases, if the operation is done early, satisfactory return of painless motion may be expected within a year. In certain injuries, however, there is so much soft part damage, especially in the anterior portion of the elbow, that bone production may occur following operation, resulting in some instances in synostosis between the radius and the ulna and causing marked limitation of function. The prognosis in operative cases should therefore be guarded.

Summary.—

Hemarthrosis, limitation of motion, and radial head tenderness characteristic signs.

Aspiration and early active motion in simple cases.

Operative removal of head in cases with displacement.

Fractures in the Neck of the Radius.—These are not as frequent as fractures of the head. In cases with gross displacement operative removal of the head is necessary. In children, however, in whom these cases are frequently seen, reduction should be done because the removal of the head fragment in the growing child will lead to a deformed joint. Reduction can occasionally be done by closed manipulation but may require open operation. Hemarthrosis will not occur if the fracture line does not run into the joint.

Separations of the Epiphysis.—If the displacement is slight a short period of immobilization with a posterior molded splint for comfort is all that is necessary. If there is sufficient hemarthrosis to cause pain aspiration should be

Injuries to the Elbow Joint

done. The splint may be removed in three or four days to be replaced by a sling until the tenderness has disappeared.

If the epiphysis has been grossly displaced one attempt at a closed reduction is justified. If this is unsuccessful operation is necessary to correct the displacement, never to remove the fragment. The operative reduction should be done as soon as possible after the injury and should be as gentle as possible to avoid further damage to the epiphyseal plate. Removal of the epiphysis will result eventually in a deformed and disabled elbow. After closed or open reduction a posterior molded splint should be applied with the elbow held at about 80 degrees for two to three weeks.

As in all injuries to the elbow in children, passive motions, forceful manipulations to increase range, and weight carrying are contraindicated, as they do more harm than good. Active use within pain limits is all the physiotherapy a child needs.

FRACTURES OF THE UPPER EXTREMITY OF THE ULNA

Fractures of the Olecranon Process.—*Occurrence.*—These are fairly common fractures in adults, not so frequent in children. They may be produced either by indirect violence or by a direct blow.

Displacement.—The proximal fragment is most frequently pulled upward by the triceps. Fractures caused by direct violence are usually stellate in type without gross displacement.

Diagnosis.—Because of the subcutaneous position of the olecranon, diagnosis of a fracture with displacement is easy. The displaced fragment is palpable and active extension of the forearm on the arm is lost. Swelling directly over the olecranon, with no palpable bony deformity, but tenderness, both direct and indirect, suggest a fracture without displacement.

Injuries to the Elbow Joint

Pathology.—In fractures caused by direct violence there is usually considerable swelling because of the damage to the overlying soft parts. The aponeurosis of the triceps, however, is intact. If there is any separation of the fragment the lateral expansion of the triceps must be torn. There may be injury to the ulnar nerve.

Treatment.—In cases where there is no displacement immobilization with a posterior molded splint, holding the elbow at right angles, is all that is necessary. The splint is for comfort and protection only and need not be worn more than a week, to be followed by a sling. Guided active motions within pain limits should be instituted early.

Where separation of the fragments has occurred, indicative of tearing of the triceps expansion, open reduction is the treatment of choice, with fixation of the fragments by wire, intramedullary pin, screws, or triceps tendon. Splint protection should be necessary for only a few days,, and active motion started early. A sling should be used for three to four weeks, but active exercises within pain limits must be encouraged.

If for some reason an operation is contraindicated the elbow can be immobilized by a posterior molded splint in complete extension. This is a very poor second-best form of treatment, but has to be resorted to in an occasional case.

Time of Immobilization.—Splints in the undisplaced fractures should be maintained for no longer than a week. Three to four weeks of immobilization is necessary when the fragments have been displaced if open reduction with internal fixation has not been carried out.

Prognosis.—Full functional return should be expected in about three months in the undisplaced and in four or five months in the operative cases. Bony union is the usual result but a dense fibrous union will give satisfactory function.

Summary.—
  Tearing of soft parts important feature in fracture with separation.

Injuries to the Elbow Joint

Treatment for undisplaced fractures, splint and guided active motion.

Treatment for displaced fractures, operative fixation.

Fractures of the Coronoid Process.—*Occurrence.*—These are relatively rare injuries, occasionally associated with posterior dislocations of the elbow. They are usually caused by a fall on the hand or forearm with the direction of force such that the coronoid is driven against the trochlea.

Displacement.—If the fragment consists of the tip of the bone it may lie free in the joint. If, however, the fracture line is more distal it may include fibers of the attachment of the brachialis and the fragment will then be pulled upward.

Diagnosis.—A painful elbow with tenderness in the antecubital fossa is suggestive of this injury. Diagnosis is usually made by x-ray examination.

Pathology.—As has been said, this injury occasionally accompanies posterior dislocation at the elbow and may be associated with considerable soft part damage and tearing of the joint capsule. On the other hand, fracture through the tip may be associated with hemarthrosis only. Where there has been tearing of the brachialis there may be an overproduction of bone in this muscle.

Treatment.—If the fragment is small, immobilization of the elbow in a semiflexed position for from two to three weeks is all that is necessary. If the fragment is large, it may be forced into place by a position of acute flexion which should be maintained about three weeks. Occasionally a small fragment will not unite and may have to be removed from the joint.

Time of Immobilization.—This is usually between two and three weeks.

Prognosis.—Functional return may be complete in three or four months. On the other hand there may be persistent limitation of motion which will require removal of the fragment. In a few cases the fragment is reattached with increase in growth, giving a mechanical block to flexion.

Summary.—

Occasionally seen with posterior dislocations.
Immobilization in flexion for from two to three weeks.

DISLOCATIONS AT THE ELBOW

Both Bones Backward.—*Occurrence.*—This is second only to dislocations of the shoulder in frequency of occurrence. In children it is the most frequent dislocation. It is usually caused by a fall on the outstretched hand, with the elbow in extension.

Displacement.—The forearm is forced backward by the mechanism of the injury and held in that position by the pull of the triceps. The coronoid usually lies behind the humerus in the olecranon fossa.

Diagnosis.—There is gross visible deformity at the elbow with the olecranon projecting posteriorly to the axis of the humerus. The relationship of the epicondyles to the olecranon is altered but that of the epicondyles to the humeral axis is unchanged, thus differentiating a dislocation from a supracondylar fracture (Fig. 50). The diagnosis should be confirmed by x-ray films because the presence of an associated fracture may not be recognized by clinical examination.

Pathology.—If the forearm is forced backward on the arm the anterior portion of the capsule must tear. There are also torn fibers of the brachialis anticus and possibly damage to the radial and median nerves, as they are stretched over the anterior aspect of the lower end of the humerus. Nerve and vessel injury are, however, rare. Because of the tearing of the anterior structures of the elbow joint the danger of myositis ossificans following a posterior dislocation is a real one.

Treatment.—Reduction should be accomplished as soon as possible in order to minimize the soft part stretching. A general anesthetic should be used for complete relaxation.

Reduction is accomplished either by hyperextension or by backward displacment of the forearm on the arm to release the coronoid from the dorsal aspect of the humerus, accompanied by steady downward traction followed by flexion. If the forearm cannot be completely flexed on the arm, reduction has not been complete and a second attempt should be made. A posterior molded splint with the elbow at right angles should be applied and maintained for three or four days for protection and rest of the soft parts. Immediate physical therapy in the form of heat and gentle massage is advisable. Active motion within pain limits may be started within two or three days in the uncomplicated cases. Extension of the forearm on the arm, however, should not be allowed for about three weeks because of the danger of redislocation.

The treatment outlined may have to be altered if there are associated fractures. Occasionally in children the epiphysis of the internal epicondyle may be pulled off at the time of the dislocation and caught in the joint as the dislocation is reduced. This complication should be recognized on postreduction x-ray films. Operation and removal of the bone from the joint with reattachment to its normal place must be done. Fractures of the radial head frequently accompany a dislocation and may necessitate an early operation as already discussed.

Time of Immobilization.—A splint is needed for physiological rest for three or four days and a sling to prevent extension should be maintained for about three weeks.

Prognosis.—In almost every case of dislocation of the elbow, follow-up x-ray plates will show calcification in the collateral ligaments. In most instances, however, the calcium deposit is not enough to interfere with function, which should be complete in from four to six months. Occasionally, however, soft part damage is so great, especially in those cases associated with fractures, that overproduction of bone results. In such cases the prognosis for full return of function should be guarded.

Summary.—

Frequent injury with characteristic posterior deformity of elbow.

Treatment by manipulative reduction under anesthesia and splint protection for from three to four days.

Soft part damage with late calcification and ossification in the tissues.

Lateral and Medial Dislocations.—These are variations of posterior dislocations and the pathology, treatment and prognosis are similar.

Forward Dislocation.—This rare injury can occur only with fracture of the olecranon. Following reduction, repair of the olecranon and triceps expansion is of primary importance.

Dislocations of the Head of the Radius.—*Occurrence.*—These injuries are almost invariably associated with a fracture of the upper third of the ulna (Monteggia fracture). With angulation or shortening of the upper ulnar shaft the radius must either dislocate or break, and it usually dislocates.

Displacement.—The displacement of the head of the radius depends on the angulation of the ulna and is usually anterior, but it may be lateral, or, rarely, posterior.

Diagnosis.—The radial head can usually be palpated anterior to its normal position. In long-standing cases this is particularly marked when the forearm is extended on the arm. In fresh injuries where the fracture of the ulna is obvious, the examiner should always look for the anterior position of the radial head. All the usual signs and symptoms of fracture are present. X-ray examination will confirm the diagnosis if it is remembered that normally a line through the long axis of the shaft of the radius will go through the capitellum (Fig. 57).

Pathology.—The head of the radius may tear through the fibers of the orbicular ligament or in some instances pull out

Injuries to the Elbow Joint

beneath it, leaving the orbicular ligament more or less intact. If the bone has torn out it may be possible to replace the head through the gap from which it emerged. Frequently, however, the torn edges of the orbicular ligament fall back and lie between the radial head and the lesser sigmoid cavity. In such instances, of course, closed reduction is impossible to maintain. Nerve and blood vessel injuries are rare.

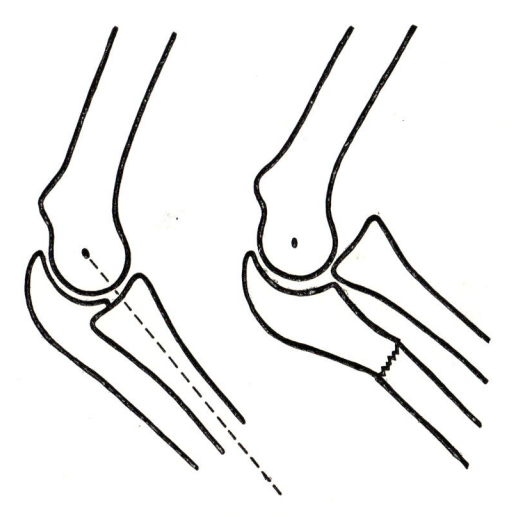

Fig. 57.

Treatment.—Closed reduction of the angulation of the ulna with the replacement of the radial head can be done in certain cases. In the majority of instances, however, it is necessary to repair the orbicular ligament at the same time that an open reduction of the ulnar fracture is accomplished. If an angular deformity of the ulna is allowed to persist, dislocation of the radius will recur. Following reduction, either closed or open, a posterior molded splint should be applied with the forearm at right angles to the arm. This should be maintained for about three weeks and followed by guided active motion.

Time of Immobilization.—A posterior molded splint should be maintained for from three to five weeks or until there is x-ray evidence of healing of the ulna.

Prognosis.—If the dislocation of the radial head is recognized early and reduced, full functional return should be expected. If the dislocation is unrecognized and allowed to persist, motions at the elbow joint will be limited. In children this limitation of motion may not occur for several years after the injury until the lower end of the humerus has increased in size to such an extent that the radial head impinges upon the lateral condyle in flexion instead of slipping by it.

Summary.—

Associated with anterior angulation or displacement of the upper ulnar shaft.

Operative repair of orbicular ligament as well as reduction of ulna usually necessary.

Closed reduction occasionally possible.

Subluxation of the Radial Head.—*Occurrence.*—This injury is found only in young children and is caused by a sudden jerk on the wrist or forearm.

Displacement.—It is supposed that the radial head is pulled slightly in the orbicular ligament, but neither clinically nor by x-ray can any displacement be made out.

Diagnosis.—Frequently the child is too young to explain his symptoms. Careful examination of the extremity, however, will elicit a sharp cry when the elbow is examined and pressure is made over the radial head. Pronation and supination of the forearm are limited. With the history that the child refuses to use the arm following a jerk or pull on the wrist, and with no pathology found elsewhere, the diagnosis is suggested. X-ray examination is of negative value only, in these cases, as it serves to rule out a fracture.

Pathology.—Very little if anything is known of the actual

Injuries to the Elbow Joint

pathology of this lesion. It is obvious by the symptomatology that some mechanical interference with rotation has occurred, *i.e.*, something has slipped out of place that can be replaced easily.

Treatment.—Firm, steady supination of the forearm while pressure is maintained over the radial head will under most circumstances relieve the condition immediately. No anesthesia is necessary. Frequently a click can be felt; many times the condition is relieved spontaneously. A sling as a protection for a few days is all that is necessary.

Time of Immobilization.—No splint is necessary. A sling may be used for a few days.

Prognosis.—Complete return of function may be expected in twenty-four hours.

Summary.—
> Caused by a jerk on hand or forearm and evidenced by pain and limitation of rotation.
>
> Reduced spontaneously or by firm supination.

Chapter 11

Injuries to the Forearm

FRACTURES OF RADIUS AND ULNA

Occurrence.—These injuries are usually seen in children and in young adults but may occur at any age. They are caused by direct or indirect violence.

Displacement.—If the fracture is in the upper third of the shaft of the radius, above the insertion of the pronator radii teres, the proximal fragment will be held supinated and flexed by the pull of the supinators. If the fracture lies below the insertion the upper fragment is likely to be in the mid-position. The original displacement is due to the direction of the fracturing force, but the pull of the flexors and extensors tends to maintain the angulation or overriding.

Diagnosis.—When there is displacement with visible deformity the diagnosis is evident. X-ray examination, however, is essential to show the obliquity or comminution of the bone ends.

Pathology.—In adults, in whom considerable violence is needed to break the bones, there is usually fairly extensive soft part damage with hemorrhage beneath the deep fascia and impairment of circulation. Cases of Volkmann's ischemic paralysis have been reported. In children, on the other hand, in whom green-stick fractures are of frequent occurrence with relatively little violence, swelling and hemorrhage may be minimal. Damage to one or more of the nerves of the forearm frequently accompanies severe injuries.

Treatment.—In children a satisfactory form of treatment is closed reduction under anesthesia followed by immobilization in plaster splints. If the fractures are in the upper third reduction can best be accomplished by supinating and flexing the lower fragment to bring it into position with the

Injuries to the Forearm

upper. The extremity is then placed in anterior and posterior molded splints which extend from the shoulder to the metacarpal heads. If the fractures are in the middle or lower third of the bones reduction can be carried out with the forearm at mid-position. Immobilization with a sugar tongs splint is satisfactory. In green-stick fractures requiring reduction both cortices should be broken through during manipulation, otherwise the deformity will tend to recur.

In adults fractures of both bones of the forearm present a problem. Reduction may be accomplished, but because of the pull of the forearm muscles adequate position is difficult to maintain. The use of Kirschner wires, one through the ulna above and one through both bones below the fracture, will aid materially in the maintenance of position. These wires should be incorporated in circular plaster after the fractures have been satisfactorily reduced. In many cases, however, open reduction with some form of internal fixation is the only way in which a satisfactory reduction can be obtained and held.

Immobilization of fractures of the shafts of the forearm bones in both adults and children should be maintained for at least eight weeks. Refractures occur with considerable frequency in this group and must be guarded against by prolonged immobilization. Finger function must therefore be stressed during the period of splinting. Persistent angulation or bowing of either bone may lead to a permanent limitation of rotation and should be avoided.

Period of Immobilization.—Splints must be maintained for at least eight weeks and sometimes longer.

Prognosis.—In children in cases where there is no angulation there is usually full functional return soon after the removal of splints. If bowing or angulation persists rotation may be permanently impaired. In adults the prognosis should be guarded.

Summary.—
  Proximal fragment supinated and flexed in fractures of the upper third of the shafts.

In children closed reduction and splints for eight weeks.
In adults Kirschner wires incorporated in plaster or operative reduction and fixation.
Anatomical restoration important to function.

FRACTURES OF A SINGLE BONE

Radius.—*Occurrence.*—Fractures of the radius most frequently occur in the lower third of the shaft and are caused either by direct or indirect violence. They are common in children.

Displacement.—The direction of the fracturing force determines to a considerable degree the angulation or overriding, but rotary displacement is largely influenced by muscle action. If the fracture line is above the insertion of the pronator radii teres the upper fragment is supinated and flexed; if below it, the upper fragment usually remains in mid-position and the lower fragment may be pronated and deviated toward the ulna. If the radius is shortened by overriding of the fragments or marked angulation, dislocation of the ulnar head occurs.

Diagnosis.—The diagnosis is usually easy because of the visible and palpable position of the bone in the distal half of the forearm.

Pathology.—There is usually less soft part damage associated with these fractures than with injuries to both bones. Nerve and large vessel lesions are rare. Delayed or nonunion is not infrequent.

Treatment.—This consists customarily of reduction and immobilization in splints. Reduction may be difficult because of the splinting action of the intact ulna and operation may occasionally be necessary. If the fracture is in the upper third of the shaft supination and flexion of the lower fragment are necessary to correct the displacement.

Time of Immobilization.—For fractures in the distal third of the bone, splint protection should be maintained for four

Injuries to the Forearm

weeks. Fractures in the middle and upper thirds should be immobilized for from six to eight weeks.

Prognosis.—Any residual deformity may result in limitation of rotation; therefore prognosis should be guarded in adults. In children full functional return is the rule.

Summary.—

Frequent injury in children.

Closed reduction and immobilization in splints usual treatment.

Anatomical correction usually necessary for complete rotation.

Ulna.—Fractures of the ulna are caused most frequently by direct violence because of the subcutaneous and vulnerable position of the shaft. As has been said before, fractures of the upper third with anterior displacement are associated with anterior dislocations of the radial head. Fractures of the middle and lower thirds can usually be reduced by manipulation and held by sugar tongs splints.

Delayed or non-union occasionally occurs and immobilization should be continued until there is evidence of bony healing.

Chapter 12

Injuries at the Wrist

FRACTURES OF THE LOWER END OF THE RADIUS

Colles' Fractures.—*Occurrence.*—Most frequent and best known of all fractures, the injury may occur at any age but is most frequently found in the older age groups. It is caused by a fall on the outstretched hand.

Displacement.—Because the fracturing force is directed upward and backward, the displacement of the lower fragment is in the same direction. This displacement may be manifested as a tilt of a few degrees merely straightening the normal volar curve of the radius, as a shift extending the entire width of the bone, or any combination of tilt and shift between these two extremes. There is usually impaction and, because the force of the trauma is up as well as back, this is frequently most marked at the dorsal cortex. The distal fragment may be in one piece or comminuted, sometimes with fracture lines into the articular surface. Shortening of the radius because of the impaction or, in rare cases, overriding, will cause a radial deviation of the hand. There may be an actual radial shift of the lower fragment. Rotation deformity may also occur. A fracture of the ulnar styloid is usually an associated lesion. In other words, a Colles' fracture may show any displacement, from an almost imperceptible angulation with no other deformity to dorsal shift and tilt, impaction, shortening and radial shift.

Diagnosis.—The normal anatomy of the wrist and the relationship of the hand to the forearm must be appreciated before deviations from the normal can be determined. A line drawn through the middle of the forearm normally meets a line drawn through the third metacarpal at the level of the wrist joint (Fig. 58). Because of the curving shape of

Injuries to the Wrist

the radial articular surface there is a slight ulnar deviation of the hand when the upper extremity hangs relaxed (Fig. 58). The volar surface of the lower radius is slightly concave, which gives a visible curve to the volar aspect of the lower third of the forearm (Fig. 59). The dorsal surface is relatively flat. The plane of the articular surface of the

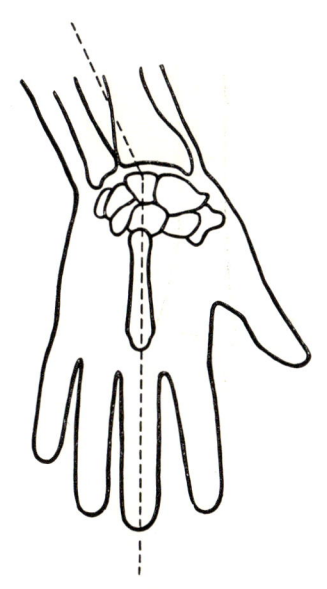

Fig. 58.—Dorsal view of normal wrist showing ulnar deviation of hand.

radius inclines slightly volarward (Fig. 59). On palpation the radial styloid is felt about 0.5 cm. distal to the ulnar styloid (Fig. 58). The dorsal surface of the lower extremity of the radius feels rough and irregular because of the grooves in the bone through which the tendons pass.

The "silver fork" deformity described in every textbook is caused by the dorsal displacement of the lower fragment. There are also usually present a radial shift or tilt of the

126   Injuries to the Wrist

hand, a loss of the volar concavity of the wrist, and a shortening of the radius with a change in the styloid relationship (Fig. 60). Where there is gross displacement the diagnosis is easy. Where there is little or no displacement the direct

Dorsal surface   *Volar surface*

Plane of articular surface

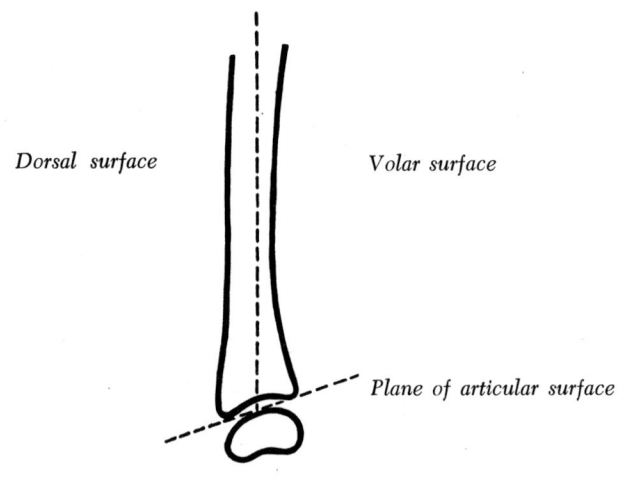

Fig. 59.—Lateral view of normal wrist.

and indirect tenderness over the lower end of the radius coupled with the history of the injury should lead the examiner to suspect a fracture. X-ray films should always be taken to show the exact nature of the injury.

Pathology.—Because the fracture is through cancellous bone the presence of comminution is of extreme importance from a standpoint of prognosis. When the fracture is reduced there may be left a wedge-shaped gap in the dorsal surface which is filled with soft bone fragments and will take long to heal. In such cases the deformity may recur if adequate protection is not maintained for a sufficient period. If shortening of the radius is allowed to persist, the relationship of the bones at the inferior radio-ulnar joint will be disturbed and may result in pain on rotation. If the distal

Injuries to the Wrist

fragment is shifted dorsally to a considerable extent there may be pressure on the median nerve and the flexor tendons as they pass over the projecting anterior end of the proximal fragment (Fig. 61). Fortunately, this complication is not

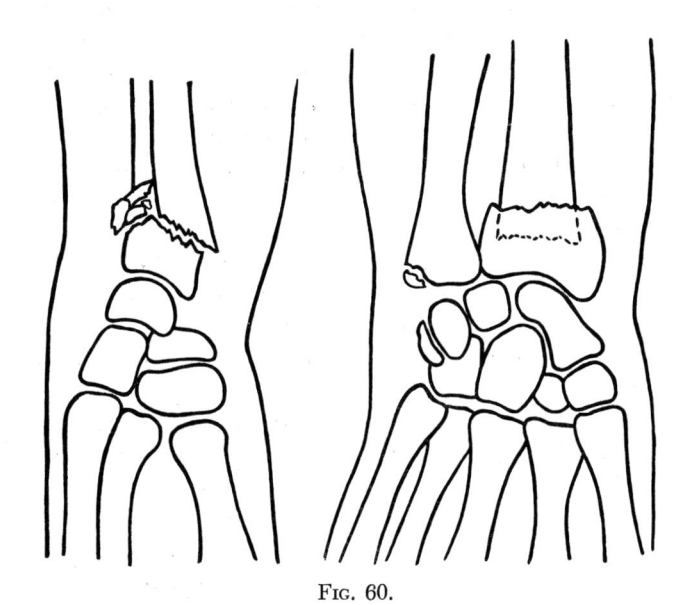

Fig. 60.

frequent, but the condition of the median nerve must always be tested. Swelling, especially of the hand and fingers, may be a distressing complication and should be combated from the initial treatment.

Treatment.—Immediate reduction under either general or local anesthesia should be done. If seen early, these fractures can be reduced very satisfactorily with the injection of novocaine into the hematoma at the fracture site. Manipulation should not be according to any set of rules but according to the needs of the individual fracture. It should be remembered that impaction must always be overcome by steady traction and a gentle rocking motion before the distal fragment can be brought forward and down into place. The shortening must be overcome by traction, the dorsal shift or angulation by pressure in a volar direction, and the radial shift by pressure on the distal fragment toward the ulna. After the fracture is reduced satisfactorily, *i.e.*, when the normal anatomical relations have been restored, it should be immobilized in some form of anterior and posterior splints. A sugar tongs splint is very satisfactory. The wrist should be placed in palmar flexion and ulnar deviation to maintain reduction. Care should be taken to flex the wrist, not the hand. Median nerve damage can occur from too acute flexion.

If there has been no displacement the acutely flexed position at the wrist is undesirable, a slight cock-up position being preferred. Where there has been gross dorsal comminution so that there is a gap in the bony structure on the dorsal surface, the time of immobilization must be prolonged. In such cases it is frequently wise to replace the splints by a plaster gauntlet after the initial swelling has gone down. Splint or gauntlet should not extend beyond the mid-palmar crease, as finger motion and use of the hand should be started from the beginning. There are certain few cases where the fragmentation is so great that the position cannot be held by splints or gauntlet. In these cases it is wise to insert two Kirschner wires, one through the bases of four medial metacarpals and one through the radius and ulna above the fracture. With traction and countertraction exerted on the wires, the fragments can be molded into position and held there while circular plaster is placed around the wrist incorporating the two wires. The wires will maintain the length of the bone during the healing period. Active motion of the fingers must be insisted on. In simple uncomplicated cases the splints should be kept on from two and a half to three weeks and then replaced by a protective wristlet for another week or two weeks. Where there has been no displacement the period may be consider-

Injuries to the Wrist

ably shortened and the patients started on hot soaks and gentle massage within the second week. In the elderly and in those cases where function is more important than ap-

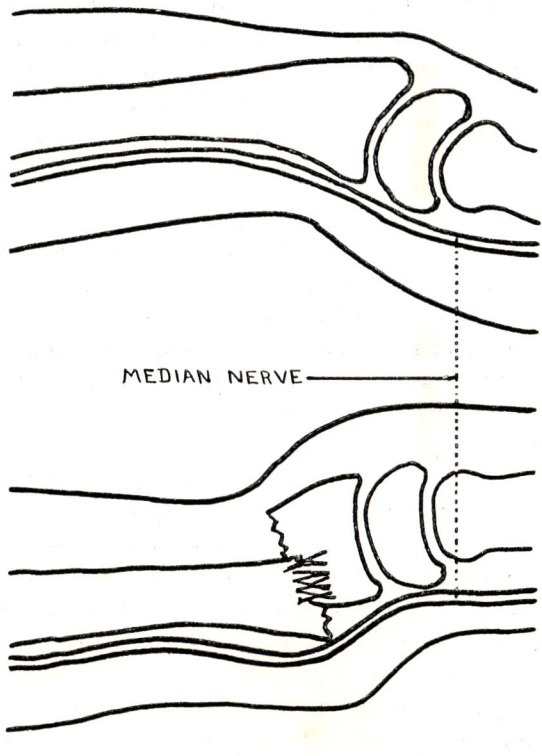

Fig. 61.

pearance, early active motion may be started from the beginning and reduction dispensed with. If there has been gross dorsal comminution it may be necessary to keep the wrist immobilized for from four to six weeks, and if wires have been used they should be kept *in situ* for six weeks.

Time of Immobilization.—Simple cases should be immobilized about two weeks, more severe types for from three to four weeks, more comminuted cases from four to six weeks, those with double wires, six weeks.

Prognosis.—Where there has been little or no displacement in a relatively young person there should be full return of function in two or three months. In the older group where there is dorsal comminution the prognosis should be guarded, for there may be residual deformity, limitation of flexion, and pain in the radio-ulnar joint on rotation.

Summary.—

The most common type of fracture.

Dorsal prominence of lower end of radius, loss of volar concavity of lower forearm, and radial tilt of hand most frequent deformities.

Early reduction and immobilization with splints.

Double Kirschner wires valuable in severely comminuted cases.

Operation rarely necessary.

Residual deformity possible source of painful motion.

Reverse Colles' Fractures.—These injuries are infrequent and are caused by a blow or fall on the dorsum of the hand, the fracturing force being directed anteriorly. The lower fragment of the radius is displaced forward and may or may not be comminuted. Reduction under anesthesia is frequently possible, and the wrist should be immobilized with the hand held in the cock-up position. A sugar tongs splint is a satisfactory means of immobilization. Some of these fractures are difficult to reduce and hold and operation may be necessary, though it offers certain technical difficulties.

Separation of Lower Radial Epiphysis.—*Occurrence.*—These are very common injuries of childhood and are caused by a fall on the outstretched hand.

Displacement.—The radial epiphysis slips posteriorly and somewhat proximally, almost invariably taking with it a wedge-shaped fragment from the posterior edge of the diaphysis (Fig. 62). The amount of displacement may be anything from 1 to 2 mm. to the entire width of the shaft.

Diagnosis.—A "silver fork" deformity at the wrist of a child suggests either an epiphyseal displacement or a fracture in the lower third of the radial shaft. Frequently an x-ray film is the only means of differentiation between the

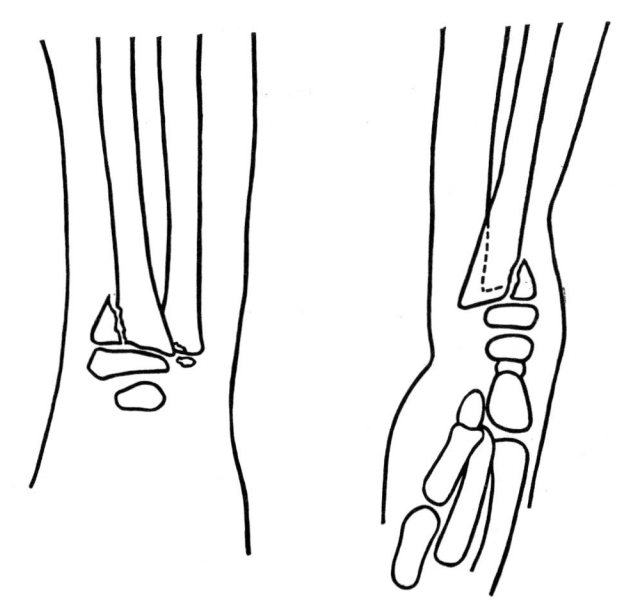

Fig. 62.—Separation of lower radial epiphysis.

two lesions. In injuries to the wrist with no resulting deformity, tenderness over the epiphyseal line, swelling and disability strongly suggest a fracture through the epiphyseal cartilage. Early x-ray plates show no evidence of such injury and the diagnosis must be made on the clinical picture. X-ray films taken two or three weeks after the injury may show a small line of subperiosteal callus extending a short distance up the shaft.

Pathology.—There is frequently not much swelling and rarely are there nerve or vessel complications. The late complication is that of growth disturbance and apparently the extent of displacement is no indication for the presence or absence of such a disturbance.

Treatment.—Reduction under an anesthetic is usually very simple if the case is seen early. Immobilization in splints for two or three weeks is all that is necessary in most cases. Where the case is seen late, open replacement of the epiphysis may be necessary in order to prevent persistent deformity. However, open reduction should only be done as a last resort, as the normal growth processes in a child will correct amazing displacements.

Time of Immobilization.—From two to three weeks.

Prognosis.—Complete functional return is usually very prompt, but growth disturbances may occur as late as two or three years after injury and the parents should always be warned of this fact. There is no known way to prevent it.

Summary.—

    Frequent injury in childhood.

    Dorsal displacement usual.

    Manipulative reduction and splints for from two to three weeks.

    Growth disturbance a possible complication.

FRACTURES OF THE CARPUS

Fractures of the Navicular (Scaphoid).—*Occurrence.*—This is the most frequently injured bone of the carpus and usually occurs in young and active adults. It is usually caused by a fall on the outstretched hand.

Displacement.—Displacement of either the distal or the proximal fragment is quite rare and occurs usually after a severe injury. Occasionally the proximal fragment may be displaced anteriorly with a dislocation of the lunate (semilunar) bone. Frequently, however, there is no displacement of either fragment.

Injuries to the Wrist

Diagnosis.—The differential diagnosis between a fracture of the navicular and a sprain of the wrist is of great importance, for a failure to recognize a fracture and immobilize it may be responsible for the development of a non-union. Characteristic signs of a fresh fracture of a navicular are swelling over the carpus, frequently with evidence of a hemarthrosis, tenderness over the navicular (especially on the volar surface), indirect tenderness elicited by pressure on the thumb upward toward the radius, pain on rocking the navicular on the radius, pain on radial deviation of the hand, limitation of flexion and extension of the wrist on the forearm. Tenderness on pressure in the anatomical snuff-box is not definite evidence of fracture unless it is more marked than the tenderness produced by similar pressure on the uninjured wrist. Characteristic signs of a sprained wrist are diffuse swelling without a hemarthrosis, generalized tenderness, usually over the dorsum of the wrist, no indirect tenderness, vague pain on rocking the navicular, quite different from the sharp pain of the fractured bone, because of the strain on the torn ligaments, and pain on ulnar deviation of the hand if the radial collateral ligament is torn.

X-ray pictures must be taken in the oblique as well as in the antero-posterior and lateral planes to show the complete bone. The hand should be so placed that the radial side is next the film. Negative x-ray films do not rule out a fracture of the navicular, and the physician must be guided by the clinical picture for his diagnosis.

Pathology.—The bone usually breaks at its mid-portion or at the junction of the middle and proximal thirds. Because of the poor blood supply of the proximal third with its lack of soft part attachments, fractures in this area frequently do not unite. The fractures in the distal third, however, almost always unite. Because of the position and character of the bone, soft part damage is usually negligible.

Treatment.—As soon as the diagnosis is made or suspected the wrist should be immobilized in a plaster-of-Paris gauntlet, extending from the mid-palmar crease to the elbow and including the proximal phalanx of the thumb. It has been found that immediate and adequate splinting affords the best chance for bony union. Immobilization of a sprain does no harm, but failure to provide early fixation for a fractured navicular may result in non-union. The wrist should be placed in slight extension to allow full use of the fingers. Abduction of the first metacarpal with slight flexion of the proximal phalanx will permit better function, which

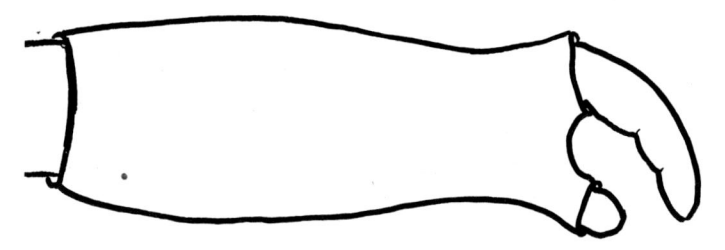

FIG. 63.—Gauntlet for navicular fracture.

should be encouraged (Fig. 63), as the gauntlet must be left in place for eight weeks at least. In fractures through the distal third the time may be cut down to four or six weeks. If, after eight weeks, x-ray films taken after the plaster has been removed show no evidence of healing further immobilization is necessary.

In order to obviate the long period of fixation various operations have been advised, bone graft, lag screw, or drilling. In selected cases, especially those that are seen several days after injury, operation may well be the treatment of choice. In late cases, where non-union has occurred, and the patient has disabling symptoms, removal of all or part of the navicular may be necessary.

Time of Immobilization.—In most cases eight weeks are necessary.

Injuries to the Wrist

Prognosis.—For cases of fractures in the middle and especially in the proximal thirds the prognosis should be guarded as to healing. Non-union of the scaphoid may give a weak and painful wrist.

Summary.—

Frequently confused with sprains of the wrist.

Diagnosis based on clinical picture.

Treatment, prolonged immobilization in plaster-of-Paris.

Non-union not uncommon in fractures of proximal third.

Fractures of the Other Carpal Bones.—Fractures of the other carpal bones are unusual, but occasionally a small chip fracture may be associated with a severe sprain. Because of the size and position of the bones they are usually seriously injured only in severe crushing accidents. Immobilization from from four to six weeks is frequently all that is necessary.

DISLOCATIONS OF THE CARPAL BONES

Dislocation of the Lunate.—*Occurrence.*—This is the most frequent dislocation of the carpal bones. It is not a common injury but should be recognized when it occurs. It is usually caused by a fall on the hyperextended hand.

Displacement.—The force of the blow drives the distal carpal bones backward and upward, widening the space between the capitate and the radius anteriorly. When the force ceases the bones slip back in place, popping the lunate out anteriorly as a watermelon seed is popped between the fingers (Fig. 64). The strong anterior radio-lunate ligament remains intact and the bone may pivot on this ligament 90 to 180 degrees (Fig. 64).

Diagnosis.—Recent cases present a swollen wrist-joint with tenderness and fulness in the anterior carpal canal. There is limitation of wrist motion and of flexion of the

136 Injuries to the Wrist

fingers. There is frequently evidence of median nerve damage because of the pressure of the lunate in the carpal canal. Late cases in which the condition has been overlooked frequently consult a doctor because of an annoying anesthesia of the fingers over the median nerve distribution. Lateral x-ray films carefully studied easily confirm the diagnosis.

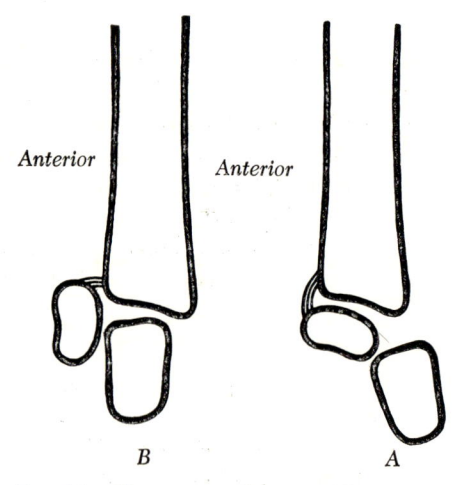

Fig. 64.—Showing mechanism of lunate dislocation.

Pathology.—The displacement of the lunate into the carpal canal causes pressure on the flexor tendons and on the median nerve, as the strong anterior carpal ligament remains intact.

Treatment.—Reduction under anesthesia should be attempted in all fresh cases. It can be accomplished by long and steady traction to separate the capitate from the radius, and extension of the hand to open up the carpo-radial joint anteriorly. At the same time, on the volar surface of the wrist, pressure is exerted from above downward and dorsally on the lunate. While traction is maintained the hand is then pulled into flexion as the lunate slips back into place. The wrist should be protected by some form of splint for about three weeks, but active use of the fingers should be encouraged. If the case is not seen early, or if reduction by closed means is not successful, open reduction should be done. In late cases removal of the bone from the carpal canal is necessary.

Time of Immobilization.—Approximately three weeks.

Prognosis.—If early reduction has been accomplished, functional return will probably be complete in a couple of months. Removal of the lunate in late cases may be followed by a weak and painful wrist.

Summary.—
  Most common carpal dislocation.
  Median nerve pressure frequent complication.
  Reduction under anesthesia treatment for early cases.
  Operative removal of bone usually best in late cases.

Chapter 13

Injuries to the Hand

FRACTURES OF THE FIRST METACARPAL

Occurrence.—This injury is most frequently produced by a badly directed blow in a fist fight and is most commonly found, therefore, in young men.

Displacement.—The fracture usually occurs at or near the base of the bone and may involve the articulation with the greater multangular (trapezium). If the joint is not involved there is an angular deformity of the shaft with the apex directly radially. If the fracture involves the joint the main fragment is displaced radially (Fig. 65). (Bennett or Stave fractures.)

Diagnosis.—Swelling of the thumb with a visible and palpable deformity at the proximal end of the first metacarpal makes the diagnosis almost certain. X-ray pictures must be taken to show the exact location and displacement of the fracture.

Pathology.—As many of these injuries involve the first metacarpo-carpal joint and are actual fracture dislocations the capsular structures are frequently torn. There is always considerable swelling but complications are almost nonexistent.

Treatment.—Fractures of the shaft with angular deformity can be corrected by manipulation and immobilized in a plaster gauntlet with the metacarpal abducted. Traction is rarely if ever necessary.

Fracture dislocations, however, though easy to reduce if seen early, are frequently difficult to hold in position without some form of continuous traction. Adhesive strips are least efficient because of their tendency to slip. A glove finger fastened to the skin by some adhesive liquid is more

Injuries to the Hand

satisfactory. Skeletal traction by means of a wire or heavy needle through the distal end of the metacarpal is probably the most efficient of all methods as the traction is exerted directly on the bone. Whatever method is used it should be attached by elastic to a firm wire banjo splint incorporated in a well-fitting plaster gauntlet with the direction of pull across the palm of the hand. The immobilizing apparatus should be kept in place for from three to four weeks.

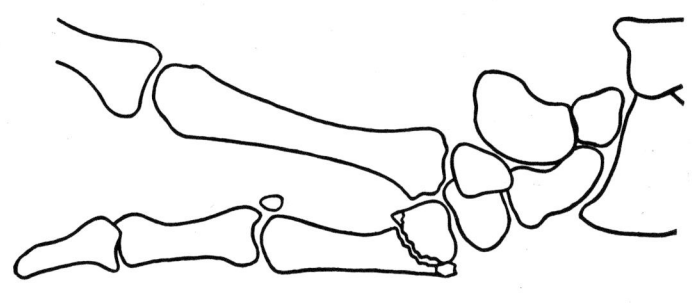

Fig. 65.

Because of the fact that traction on thumb or finger for any prolonged period results in a stiffened joint requiring months to regain motion, it has been used less and less. In some cases excellent functional results can be obtained by maintaining position as well as possible by a simple splint for only a few days, followed by hot soaks and active motion.

It should always be remembered in dealing with any injuries of the thumb that its opposing action is of vital importance. Therefore, it should never be immobilized in full abduction for any length of time if there is any danger of ankylosis. A stiff first metacarpo-carpal joint in abduction makes the thumb an almost useless member.

Time of Immobilization.—Three to four weeks if traction is used, preferably less.

Prognosis.—Functional results usually satisfactory.

Summary.—
  Injury received in a fight.
  Radial displacement of distal fragment.
  Traction necessary in fracture dislocations.
  Prognosis usually good.

FRACTURES OF THE OTHER METACARPALS

Occurrence.—These fractures are of frequent occurrence in young adult life by either direct or indirect violence. Fighting is frequently a cause.

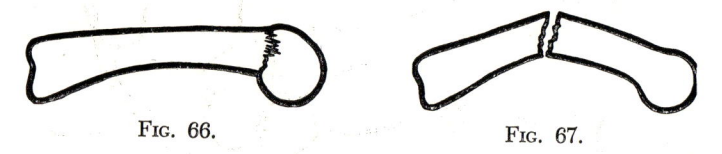

Fig. 66.

Fig. 67.

Displacement.—Fractures at the neck of the metacarpal with anterior tilt of the head are common (Fig. 66). Transverse fractures may occur in the shaft with dorsal displacement or angulation and are due to direct violence (Fig. 67). Spiral or oblique fractures of one bone usually show little or no displacement due to the splinting action of the intact metacarpals. If two or more are broken shortening and angulation are characteristic. Fractures at the base of the metacarpals are rarely displaced.

Diagnosis.—Because of the ease of palpation of the bones on the dorsum of the hand the diagnosis of fracture of the metacarpal is usually obvious. Fractures of the base where the deformity is minimal are more difficult to diagnose, but should be suggested by direct and indirect tenderness and swelling. X-ray examination is essential.

Pathology.—Swelling is apt to be considerable and in injuries caused by crushing may reach such proportions as to threaten the blood supply of the fingers.

Injuries to the Hand

Treatment.—Fractures of the neck should be reduced if the anterior displacement of the head is sufficient to interfere with grip. Because of the small distal fragment they are frequently difficult to manipulate and a small Thomas wrench or similar instrument may be necessary. Strong pressure on the proximal phalanx as it is flexed to 90 degrees on the metacarpal may reduce a fresh fracture. Following

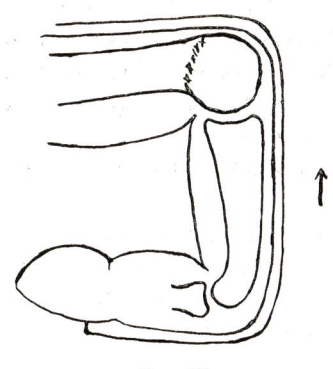

Fig. 68.

reduction the position should be maintained by a plaster splint holding the finger flexed to 90 degrees on the hand (Fig. 68). This should be maintained for about three weeks during which period active use of the other fingers should be encouraged. Fractures of the neck of the fifth metacarpal are of importance from a cosmetic point of view primarily, as the resulting dropped knuckle may not be considered esthetic. From a functional standpoint it can usually be disregarded and treated by early active motion.

Transverse fractures of a single metacarpal can usually be reduced by manipulation and held by a molded plaster splint with the hand in moderate flexion. Oblique fractures with little or no displacement may be protected by a molded splint in flexion until the acute pathology has subsided, followed by active motion within pain limits. The earlier function is restored the better the result.

If there is gross displacement of two or more metacarpals and position cannot be obtained by manipulative reduction, operation with internal fixation by intramedullary pins, small screws, or plates will usually give excellent results, as this method allows active use of the fingers almost immediately. The use of skeletal traction has been widely discarded because of the impaired function of the fingers. Function should never be sacrificed for anatomy.

Fractures of the base of the metacarpals should be given protection for a few days only and then treated by hot soaks and active motion.

Bony union usually takes place in from four to six weeks in shaft fractures.

Time of Immobilization.—Four weeks.

Prognosis.—If there has been little or no displacement and active motion has been started early, full use of the hand should be reached in four to six weeks.

Summary.—
  Frequent injuries.
  Displacement of neck fractures, forward tilting of head.
  Displacement of shaft fractures, angulation with apex dorsally; frequent overriding.
  Manual reduction and immobilization or operation.

FRACTURES OF THE PHALANGES

Occurrence.—These injuries are frequent especially in manual laborers. They may be caused by any of the common mishaps of every-day life: a slamming door, an ill-directed hammer or an unguarded machine.

Displacement.—If the fracture is in the shaft of the proximal phalanx there is usually anterior angulation. If the distal phalanx is injured a crush of the tuft usually results.

Injuries to the Hand

Diagnosis.—The deformity may be apparent but swelling may mask it and x-rays should always be taken if direct and indirect tenderness suggest a fracture.

Pathology.—A blow on the distal phalanx may give rise to a painful subungual hematoma. Fractures at a joint will cause periarticular swelling which may last many months.

Treatment.—Displaced fractures of the proximal phalanx must be reduced to prevent interference with the flexor tendon. This can usually be accomplished by manipulation and the position held by a splint with the finger in moderate flexion. If there is an oblique fracture with overriding which cannot be held in position traction by means of a pin through the pulp may be necessary. Traction through the nail is uncomfortable and Japanese basket-weave splints unsafe.

Fingers should be immobilized in slight flexion, never more than the injured finger, and always for as short a time as possible. A stiff finger may cost a skilled workman his economic life.

Chip fractures around a joint should be protected by a curved splint for a few days only and then be treated by hot soaks and active exercise.

Fractures of the distal phalanx are usually of less importance than the resulting hematoma. A drill hole through the nail to release the underlying blood is usually all the treatment indicated.

"Baseball fingers" or avulsion of the extensor tendon with or without a chip fracture of the distal phalanx should be immobilized with the terminal joint hyperextended and the proximal joint flexed at 90 degrees for at least six weeks. The prognosis is good if the position is maintained long enough.

Time of Immobilization.—As short as possible.

Prognosis.—Good if active function can be started early, guarded if traction is necessary.

Summary.—
  Common injuries of every-day life.
  Immobilization in moderate flexion.
  Early active motion as soon as possible.
  Prognosis usually good.

DISLOCATIONS OF THE METACARPALS AND PHALANGES

Dislocations of the Metacarpo-phalangeal Joints.—Dislocations of the first metacarpo-phalangeal joint are sometimes

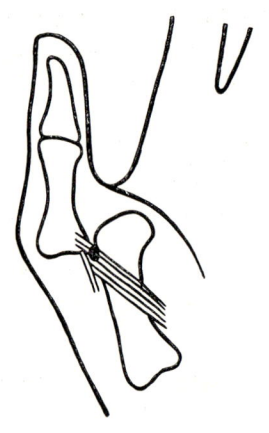

Fig. 69.—Complex dislocation of the thumb.

complicated. A complex or complete dislocation occurs when the metacarpal head slips anteriorly between the heads of the flexor brevis; the volar portion of the capsule, which is thickened and fibrocartilaginous (glenoid ligament), tears from the metacarpal and drops between the phalanx and the metacarpal head (Fig. 69). The long flexor tendon will slip to one side or the other of the metacarpal. The deformity is obvious, but the reduction may be very difficult if not impossible by closed means. Hyper-

Injuries to the Hand

extension of the thumb with traction and a kind of "milking" motion, in an attempt to slip the interposed capsule over the head of the metacarpal, may sometimes reduce the dislocation. Usually open reduction is necessary. Immobilization in slight flexion for about ten days following reduction is wise. The motion in this joint following open reduction is sometimes quite limited but does not seem to be a handicapping disability.

Dislocations of the other metacarpo-phalangeal joints are less frequently seen. Because of the thickened volar portion of the capsule (glenoid ligament), which is loosely attached to the metacarpal but firmly attached to the phalanx, they present to a somewhat slighter degree the same problem as do the dislocations of the thumb. If the capsule slips between the phalanx and the metacarpal, reduction by closed means may be very difficult and accomplished only by hyperextension, traction, and a "milking" motion to force the interposed capsule out of the joint. Flexion as a means of reduction is dangerous for it may convert a simple into a complex dislocation.

Dislocations of Interphalangeal Joints.—These dislocations are easily recognized and almost as easily reduced by manual traction if seen early. Immobilization by some simple splint for about ten days is all that it necessary. X-ray films should be made to rule out small fractures.

Part III. The Trunk

Chapter 14

Injuries to the Chest

FRACTURES OF THE RIBS

THESE injuries are of frequent occurrence and are usually caused by direct violence, such as a fall against the edge of a bathtub or against a projecting door. They may occur spontaneously after prolonged and violent coughing. A fracture of a single rib is rarely displaced. If several ribs are broken there may be overriding with or without tearing of the pleura and the lung tissue. The diagnosis is suggested by the history, by pain on inspiration and cough, by direct tenderness at the site of injury and by indirect tenderness produced by compression of the thoracic cage. Treatment consists of circumferential strapping of the chest with wide adhesive strips over flannel. If several ribs are broken and if overriding is present strapping is contraindicated as it will increase the displacement. Novocaine injection of the intercostal nerves or a paravertebral block will greatly relieve the pain and increase the comfort of the patient. Hemothorax and pneumothorax are not uncommon complications of multiple rib fractures and should be treated symptomatically with aspiration as indicated. Uncomplicated rib fractures usually heal in three weeks and non-union is extremely rare.

Chapter 15

Injuries to the Spine

First Aid Treatment.—The initial care of the patient with a spine injury is of paramount importance. Injudicious handling may cause irremedial damage to the spinal cord. Any person complaining of pain in the back following an accident should always be lifted face down to prevent flexion of the spine. The usual practice of lifting a person by hips and shoulders allowing the spine to jack-knife should never be permitted. The injured person should be rolled "all in one piece" on to his face on to a stretcher, a rug or a board so that extension of the spine is maintained until the extent of damage has been ascertained.

FRACTURES OF THE VERTEBRAL BODY

Occurrence.—This not uncommon injury is caused by any violence producing a sudden flexion or jack-knifing of the spinal column.

Displacement.—Characteristically the involved vertebra is wedged anteriorly (Fig. 70). Compression of the entire body is less common. The usual site of injury is at the junction of the dorsal and lumbar curves, *i.e.,* the twelfth dorsal or first or second lumbar, though it may occur at any level.

Diagnosis.—Any accident producing sudden flexion of the spine such as a fall from a height on the heels or buttocks, a weight falling on the shoulders as in a mine cave-in, even a severe jolt in a car may cause a compression fracture of a vertebral body. The symptoms may be mild and the patient able to go about his daily activities with only a mild backache. Tenderness directly over the spinous process of the

Injuries to the Spine

involved vertebra with some protective muscle spasm should suggest the diagnosis. In severe crushing a palpable kyphosis may be present or a loss of the normal lumbar curve. Confirmatory x-ray films must be taken in the lateral as well as the antero-posterior plane as frequently the latter will not show the lesion clearly.

Pathology.—The strong anterior vertebral ligament remains intact in these lesions. Nerve root signs are infrequent but may be manifested as girdle pains. In the more severe type of injury a retroperitoneal hematoma may give rise to abdominal signs and symptoms closely resembling those of a ruptured viscus. Even in the milder group abdominal distention may be a distressing complication. Fractures of the posterior vertebral elements occasionally are associated with compression fractures of the body and should not be overlooked. Fractures accompanied by serious cord lesions will be discussed separately.

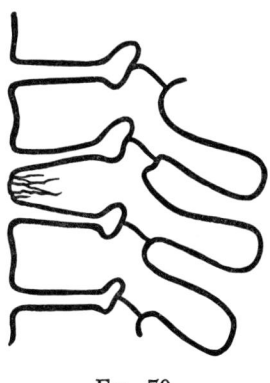

Fig. 70.

Treatment.—In recent fractures of the lower dorsal or lumbar vertebræ correction of the anterior wedging can be accomplished by hyperextension of the spine which causes a fanning out of the intact anterior ligament. This can be done by several methods, the most satisfactory of which exert some form of traction on the spinal column as well as hyperextension. The patient may be placed prone on a table with his ankles attached by a rope to a pulley in the ceiling or on a frame. As his legs and pelvis are gradually lifted by traction on the rope his spine is slowly extended. He may be placed supine over a frame which is gradually raised to extend his back, the weight of his legs acting as traction. Or he may be placed supine on a reversed Gatch bed, the knee portion of which is raised to allow extension of the spine (Fig. 71). Whatever method is used lateral x-ray pictures should be taken to check the reduction. If this is satisfactory a well-fitting plaster jacket should be immediately applied extending anteriorly from the suprasternal notch to the symphysis pubis and covering the lower dorsal and lumbar region behind (Fig. 72). As soon as possible

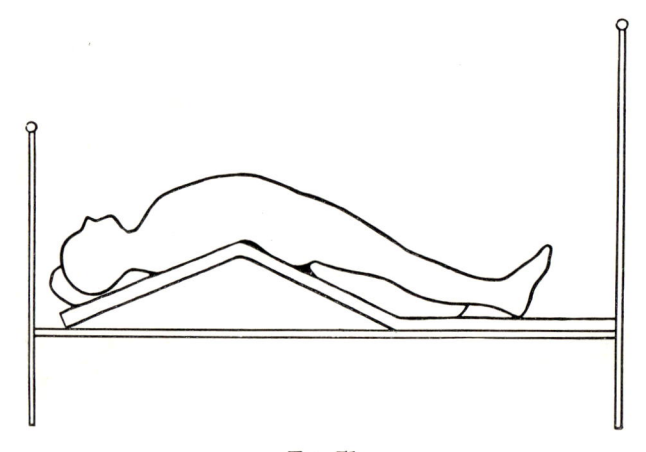

Fig. 71.

the patient should become ambulatory and be instructed in back strengthening exercises. The plaster jacket should remain in place for from eight to ten weeks. In severe injuries it may be wise to fit the patient with a Taylor spine brace for another two to three months. In mild compressions such protection is not necessary.

In elderly people such a regimen may be unwise and rest in bed for a few days followed by a Taylor brace protection may be all the treatment indicated. The same procedure is satisfactory for the upper dorsal vertebræ where correction by hyperextension is almost impossible due to the relative immobility of the thoracic spine.

Injuries to the Spine

Time of Immobilization.—Eight weeks in plaster.

Prognosis.—In those cases where the diagnosis has been made early and treatment promptly instituted the prognosis should be good. In late cases where correction has not been obtained weakness and backache may persist. Spinal fusion may be necessary.

Summary.—

> A frequent back injury caused by sudden flexion of the trunk.
>
> Diagnosis suggested by backache and tenderness over the affected vertebra, confirmed by lateral x-ray plates.
>
> Treatment, hyperextension and immobilization in a plaster jacket for eight weeks.

Fractures With Cord Injury.—These cases, caused by serious trauma, demand expert care. Careful reduction of the bony deformity at the earliest possible moment is essential because the correction of the deformity may relieve the pressure on the cord. If the cord has been completely severed or crushed, the general care of the patient to avoid bed-sores and bladder infection is the first consideration. If however, the paralysis is due to pressure on the cord by displaced bone, reduction may relieve the symptoms. In certain cases laminectomy is indicated for the relief of pressure.

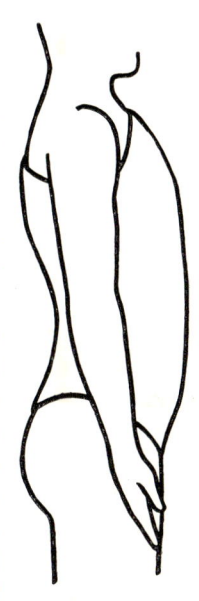

Fig. 72.

FRACTURES OF THE TRANSVERSE PROCESS

The transverse processes are surrounded front and back by large muscles and have muscle fibers attached to them. They are not weight-bearing structures. Fractures may be produced either by direct violence, like a blow or a kick, or by sudden muscle strain. They cannot be broken without considerable soft part damage, *i.e.*, extensive muscle bruising and tearing with hemorrhage. The bone injury is negligible and treatment should be directed at the soft tissue.

Rest in bed for a few days with heat, gentle massage and exercise within pain ylimits is all that is required. The patient should be told how insignificant the fracture is and exercise within pain limits is all that is required. The muscle damage is repaired. Immobilization in a plaster jacket is not only unnecessary but unwise as it allows the formation of fibrous tissue in the inactive muscles with a prolonged disability period as a result.

DISLOCATIONS OF THE VERTEBRÆ

Dislocations with or without fracture occur most frequently in the cervical region because of the wide range of motion normally found there. Diving accidents are among the most frequent causes. Complete or partial paralysis may be immediate. The head is held forward and may be tilted. The mobility of the neck is greatly limited. X-ray pictures are essential to ascertain the extent of the bone damage. Reduction must be done without delay to reduce the pressure on the spinal cord. Manipulation under an anesthetic, if necessary, should only be attempted by an expert as it is hazardous. Traction on the head, with extension of the neck, must be maintained throughout the maneuver. A safer method is that of skeletal traction by means of tongs or wires in the skull. The head of the bed is raised so that the body provides counter-traction. Frequent x-ray checks are necessary. Traction by means of a head halter under chin and occiput is less efficient but can be used if necessary. After reduction has been accomplished a plaster cuirass should be applied to maintain position. This should be left on for eight weeks and fol-

Injuries to the Spine

lowed by a leather collar for six months. In all injuries to the cervical vertebræ x-ray pictures taken through the open mouth are essential to show the odontoid process. An undetected fracture here, even though undisplaced, is a source of great danger to the patient if it is not immobilized while it is uniting. In such an injury, unprotected, a sudden jerk of the head may cause displacement and instantaneous death.

Fracture dislocations elsewhere in the spinal column are fortunately infrequent in civilian practice. They are caused by violent accidents and should be reduced immediately by traction and the necessary manipulation. Cord damage is frequent.

Incomplete dislocations or subluxations of the cervical vertebræ are common. They are caused by a sudden twist of the neck, usually when the muscles are not "on guard." The patient presents a characteristic picture; the head is tilted to one side and held stiffly. Pain is not usually a presenting symptom. The head can be tilted further but cannot be straightened beyond the midline. The muscles of the long side of the neck are in spasm and tenderness can usually be elicited on that side of one of the cervical vertebræ posteriorly. Stereoscopic x-ray films taken in the lateral plane will show a slight upward shift of one articular facet on its neighbor. Head traction manually or by head halter will reduce a recent lesion relatively quickly. Relaxation of the muscle spasm by anesthetic alone will often effect a reduction. Prolonged head traction may be necessary in those cases where the displacement has existed for some time. Following reduction in the early case a Shantz collar for two or three days is all that is necessary. In the more stubborn cases where reduction has been difficult longer protection by means of a plaster collar for two to three weeks may be advisable.

Chapter 16

Injuries to the Pelvic Girdle

FRACTURES OF THE ILIUM

FRACTURES of the wing or ala of the ilium are relatively rare and are almost always caused by direct violence. Deformity does not usually result in disability so treatment should be directed to the associated soft part damage. Rest in bed and physical therapy to hasten the absorption of extravasated blood are usually all that is required.

Either the superior- or the inferior-anterior spine may be avulsed by sudden muscle action. Treatment consists either of bed-rest with the thigh held flexed on the trunk or of a short plaster spica with the thigh in flexion. Operative replacement of the fragment with internal fixation may be used to shorten the period of disability.

FRACTURES OF THE ISCHIUM AND PUBIS

Fractures of a single ramus are not displaced due to the splinting action of the intact ramus. The diagnosis is suggested by direct and indirect tenderness and confirmed by x-ray. Bed-rest from ten days to two weeks is all the treatment required. Crutches should be used until weight-bearing is painless.

If two or more rami are fractured the problem is far more serious. These injuries are usually the result of a severe crushing accident and may be associated with bladder or urethral damage. The patient may be in severe shock depending on the extent of the soft part damage. Palpation of the pubic region will elicit tenderness and may reveal bony irregularity. Lateral compression of the iliac crests

Injuries to the Pelvic Girdle 155

will produce indirect tenderness. All patients with pelvic injury should be immediately investigated for evidence of bladder injury and the urine examined for the presence of

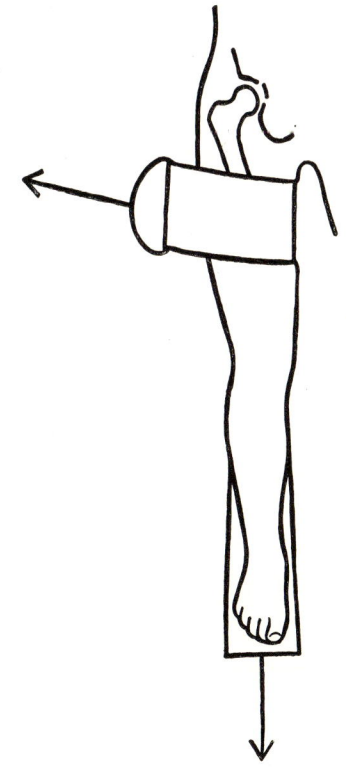

Fig. 73.

red blood cells. Bladder or urethral injury, if present, is of primary importance.

If the bone ends are overriding no form of compression bandage should be used as this will only increase the displacement. Traction on the lower extremities with a canvas sling supporting the pelvis may be satisfactory (Fig. 73).

If there is a trapdoor type of displacement or wide separation at the symphysis associated with displacement at one sacro-iliac joint, reduction may be accomplished by sling compression of the pelvis with traction on the affected leg. Watson-Jones advocates reduction by manipulation with the patient lying on the uninjured side followed by immobilization in a plaster spica. Traction or immobilization should be maintained from six to eight weeks. The ultimate prognosis is usually good for bony union and return of function. In women of child-bearing age, or younger, restitution of the shape of the pelvis is important because of possible interference with child-birth.

FRACTURES OF THE ACETABULUM

These injuries are frequently caused by a blow against the greater trochanter. If undisplaced they can be treated by suspension of the extremity with light traction and active motion in the apparatus within pain limits. Weight-bearing should not be allowed for eight weeks.

If the fragments are displaced, traction outward on the femoral head by means of a wire through the greater trochanter or a screw inserted into it may pull the fragments into place. (See Central Dislocations of the Hip, p. 172.) Operative reduction is extremely difficult. Active motion within pain limits should be instituted early but weight-bearing delayed for at least twelve weeks.

The prognosis should be guarded as traumatic arthritis and late degenerative changes in the femoral head may result.

Part IV. The Lower Extremity

Chapter 17

Injuries at the Hip Joint

FRACTURES OF THE UPPER EXTREMITY OF THE FEMUR

Intracapsular Fractures.—*Occurrence.*—These injuries are seen most commonly in the elderly, particularly in old women. They are usually caused by some mild trauma like falling on a slippery floor or tripping on a step. They are rarely seen in young adults.

Displacement.—If the fracture is caused by indirect violence as by a twisting force the distal fragment is usually externally rotated and displaced upward on the head with adduction of the shaft producing a varus deformity (Fig. 74). The neck fragment may lie in front of the head with the fractured surface of the head lying against the side of the neck. There may be some impaction if the violence is direct, *i.e.*, a fall on the greater trochanter; the fragments may be impacted with little or no displacement or in a valgus position.

Diagnosis.—Every individual of middle age or over who complains of pain in the hip following a fall however trivial should be considered to have a fracture until proved otherwise. The fact that the patient was able to walk after the accident does not necessarily rule out a broken hip. If there is displacement the diagnosis is relatively simple. Marked external rotation, shortening of the extremity compared to the opposite side as measured from anterior-superior iliac spine to the medial malleolus, pain on attempted motions

158 Injuries to the Hip Joint

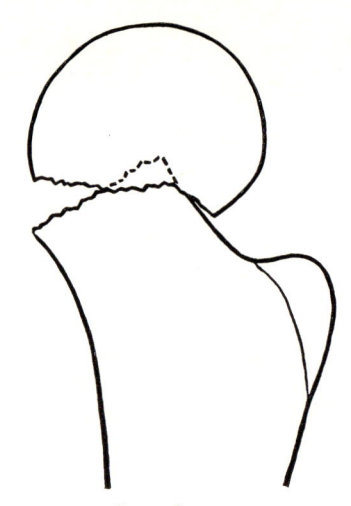

Lateral view

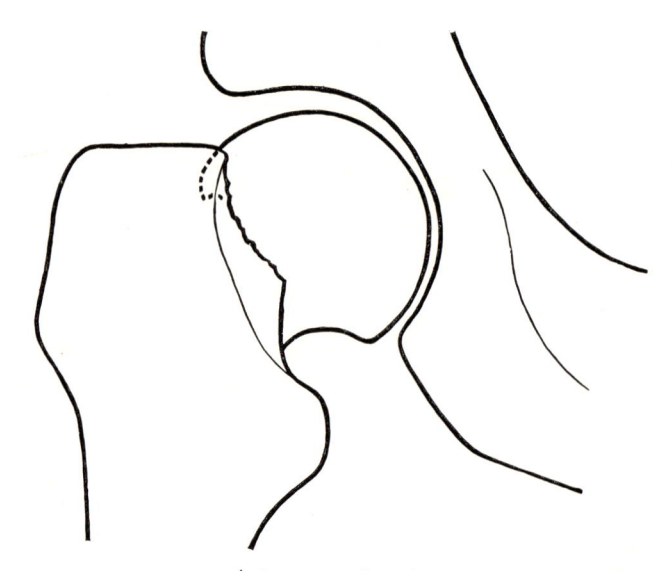

Antero-posterior view

Fig. 74.

Injuries to the Hip Joint

of the hip and indirect tenderness elicited by tapping the heel are the cardinal signs. Two other signs of little more than academic interest are Nelaton's line and Bryant's triangle. Nelaton's line extends from the anterior-superior spine to the ischial tuberosity, passing normally through the tip of the greater trochanter. If the neck of the femur is

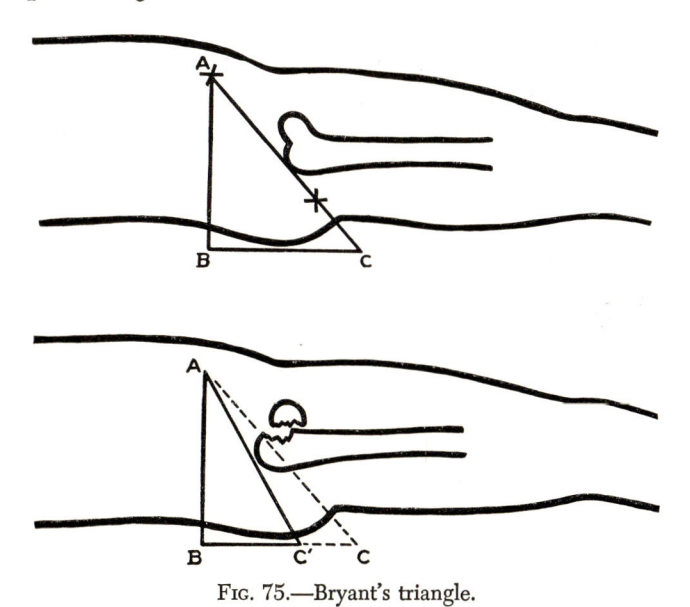

Fig. 75.—Bryant's triangle.

broken with coxa vara displacement of the fragments, the tip of the greater trochanter will be above the line. Bryant's triangle is formed by a line dropped from the anterior-superior spine perpendicular to the table with the patient supine and by a line from the anterior-superior spine through the tip of the greater trochanter with the table as the base. A comparison of the two sides will show that the base on the affected side is shorter (Fig. 75).

If the fracture is impacted and in valgus position there may be no shortening and no external rotation; the range of motion may be only slightly limited and indirect tenderness equivocal. In spite of negative clinical evidence, the history of a fall in an older person with some pain and disability in the hip makes the taking of roentgenograms in antero-posterior and lateral views an obligation. If an impacted fracture of the hip is missed and the patient allowed to walk prematurely, disimpaction and displacement will occur.

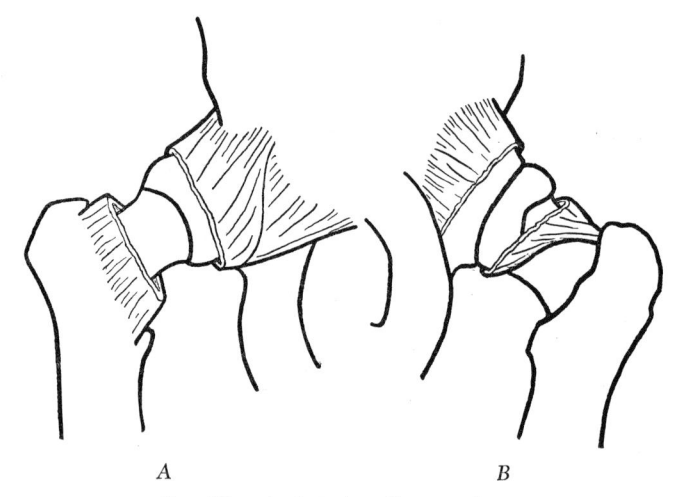

FIG. 76.—*A*, Anterior; *B*, posterior.

Pathology.—The capsule of the hip joint is attached anteriorly to the intertrochanteric line and posteriorly to the outer third of the neck (Fig. 76). There is, therefore, a considerable portion of the neck which is entirely intracapsular and obtains its blood supply from the synovial vessels and from the vessels in the bone running in from the shaft. The head receives part of its circulation from the vessels entering it by way of the ligamentum teres. The nearer the fracture line is to the head the greater is the chance for non-union.

Injuries to the Hip Joint

Treatment.—The correction of any existing displacement and the maintenance of that correction until healing has occurred are the ends toward which any form of treatment must be directed. Because of the great danger of non-union the fractured surfaces must be brought into close apposition and held there as firmly as possible. Reduction is accomplished by strong traction until the shortening is overcome (checked by comparative measurements), by direct outward pull to disengage the fragments, by internal rotation to correct the external rotation (checked by the amount of internal rotation possible in the normal leg) and by abduction to hold the reduced fracture in position (checked by the limit of abduction in the normal extremity). If the reduction is attempted with the extremity extended, either an assistant is necessary to exert traction while the operator is manipulating the thigh, or a fracture table with mechanical traction must be used. By means of the Leadbetter maneuver the operator alone can do the reduction satisfactorily. With the hip and knee flexed to right angles, and the leg over the operator's shoulder, upward pull of considerable force can be exerted on the hip. Outward leverage, internal rotation and abduction can be accomplished as the knee is forced inward and the extremity extended and abducted. If the heel of the extended leg is then balanced in the operator's palm, the foot will remain upright if adequate internal rotation and impaction have been secured (Leadbetter's sign). If the foot swings gradually into external rotation, impaction in satisfactory position has not been obtained. The position of the fracture should be immediately checked by x-ray films in two positions. Immobilization of the reduced fracture can be accomplished by a well-fitting plaster spica extending from the axillæ to the toes on the affected side (Fig. 77), or a shorter spica from the waist to the knee of the normal leg and the toes of the injured extremity (Fig. 78). Immobilization must be maintained for a minimum of eight weeks, usually from twelve to sixteen weeks. During that period the patient must be turned on her face at least twice a day and her skin given scrupulous care to avoid the distressing complication of pressure sores.

Because such prolonged immobilization is a threat to the life of the elderly, in most hospitals now some form of internal fixation has taken the place of the external plaster-of-Paris spica. The most efficient and most widely used is the three-flanged vitallium nail described by Smith-Petersen. This may be inserted through a relatively small incision over the outer side of the trochanteric region after a closed reduction has been performed. However, an open reduction with the insertion of the nail by direct vision gives a more

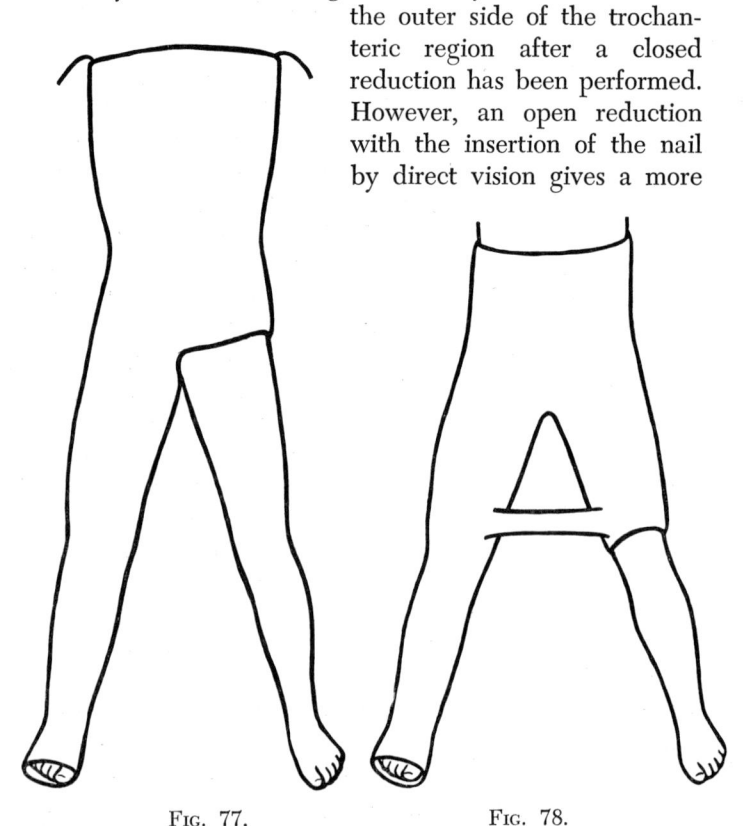

Fig. 77.   Fig. 78.

Injuries to the Hip Joint

accurate apposition of the fragments and seems to add little to the risk to the patient if properly carried out by an experienced surgeon. Whether the reduction is closed or open, the sooner it is done after injury the better for the patient. Following fixation by internal means, pin, nail, or screw, the patient is allowed in a chair as soon as possible, within a day or two, and permitted to walk with crutches as soon as her strength permits, without putting weight on the injured leg. By this regimen many of the complications associated with the previous treatment of fractured hips have been greatly diminished.

Impacted fractures of the neck of the femur in valgus position will heal with bony union in most instances. In these cases the fracture line is not subjected to cross strain and weight-bearing in a walking plaster spica may be allowed. Fixation by a nail through the fracture to prevent disimpaction will allow the patient full activity though weight-bearing should not be allowed for from six to eight weeks.

Time of Immobilization.—When plaster is used the period may be anywhere from eight to twenty weeks, usually twelve to fourteen. In all instances no weight-bearing should be allowed for at least six months with the exception of impacted fractures in valgus as noted above.

Prognosis.—No form of treatment as yet devised will prevent the complication of early aseptic necrosis of the head or the development of slow degenerative changes which may appear two or three years after the fracture has apparently healed by bony union. The prognosis should, therefore, always be guarded. Non-union will occur in a certain percentage of cases but less frequently when accurate reduction has been obtained.

Summary.—

- A frequent injury in elderly women following slight trauma.
- Characteristic deformity, external rotation and shortening of the extremity.

Treatment, reduction and immobilization by a plaster spica or by internal fixation, preferably the Smith-Petersen nail.

No weight-bearing for at least six months except in special group of impacted valgus cases.

Delayed and non-union not infrequent, therefore guarded prognosis.

Intertrochanteric Fractures.—*Occurrence.*—These injuries occur in about the same age group as the preceding, possibly somewhat younger. They are caused by a fall, usually directly on the thigh.

Displacement.—There is usually shortening in intertrochanteric fractures and there may be adduction of the distal fragment. External rotation of the extremity may be present (Fig. 79).

Diagnosis.—As shortening, external rotation and indirect tenderness are usually present in both types of fracture it is frequently difficult to distinguish an intertrochanteric from a femoral neck fracture. In the former, ecchymosis and a visible angular deformity with swelling in the trochanteric area are usually present due to the concomitant soft part damage. X-ray studies are essential.

Pathology.—Because of the excellent blood supply and the mass of soft parts surrounding this area, bony union is the rule rather than the exception. It has been said that these fractures heal regardless of the treatment.

Treatment.—Reduction can usually be readily accomplished by traction sufficient to restore length and moderate internal rotation. Maintenance of reduction by some form of traction, either by means of a Steinman pin through the supracondylar area of the femur or by Russell traction is satisfactory. A plaster spica is suitable in many instances. However, both these methods necessitate prolonged inactivity for the patient with the usual systemic complications of prolonged bed stay for the elderly. Therefore internal fixation by some means, a Smith-Petersen pin (Fig. 80), a

Injuries to the Hip Joint

Lorenzo or lag screw fastened to a lateral plate, or an angled pin and plate device is the treatment of choice, as it allows the patient to be out of bed. As many of these fractures are comminuted, some form of lateral plate is usually necessary to prevent a varus deformity. Weight-bearing

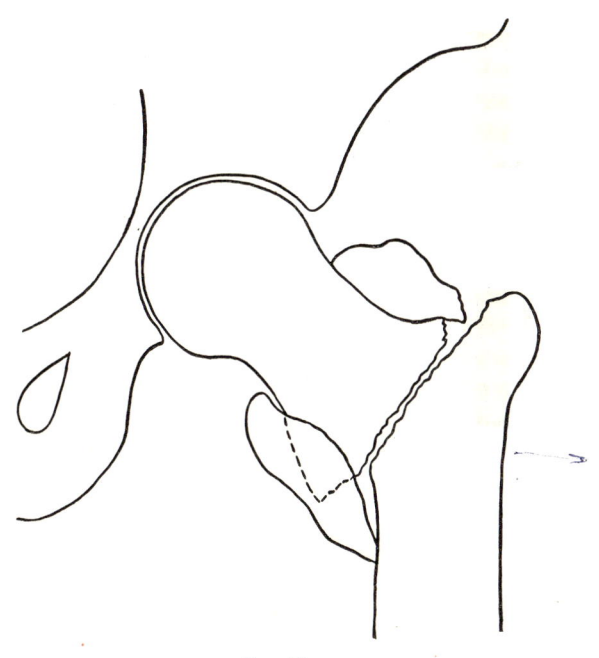

Fig. 79.

can be permitted much earlier than in intracapsular fractures, because of the better healing, usually within three months.

In the very elderly whose condition does not warrant operation, and who cannot safely remain in bed, stabilization of the legs by Wilkie boots or Roger Anderson's "Well leg traction" apparatus will allow the patient to be moved into a chair with relative comfort.

Time of Immobilization.—The plaster or the traction should be maintained for about eight weeks.

Prognosis.—These fractures usually heal with excellent bone repair and adequate function. Occasionally a coxa vara deformity will persist with slight shortening and limitation of hip motion.

Summary.—

  Similar in signs to intracapsular fractures plus evidence of soft tissue damage.

  Treatment by reduction and continued traction or plaster spica for eight weeks or by internal fixation and early active motion without weight-bearing.

  Bony union the rule.

Subtrochanteric Fractures.—*Occurrence.*—These injuries in civilian life are less frequent than the preceding and are usually caused by severe violence. They occur in active adults.

Displacement.—The upper fragment is adducted and externally rotated. It is also flexed if the lesser trochanter is still attached to it. The lower fragment is adducted and pulled upward. Shortening is usually marked and an angulation with its apex outward is visible (Fig. 81).

Diagnosis.—The shortening of the extremity is usually marked but as it takes place below the tip of the greater trochanter, Nelaton's line and Bryant's triangle remain unchanged (Fig. 82). Evidences of soft part damage are usually present and the deformity can frequently be palpated if the swelling is not too great. A false point of motion is apparent on any motion of the extremity.

Pathology.—Because of the usual mechanism, *i.e.*, severe trauma, these fractures are apt to be comminuted and to be accompanied by considerable soft part damage. Healing occurs with a large mass of soft callus which will allow angulation if the fracture site is not protected for a long period.

Injuries to the Hip Joint

Treatment.—Because of the position of the upper fragment in external rotation, abduction and flexion, the lower fragment must also be externally rotated, abducted and flexed. This can be accomplished and maintained by skeletal traction in what was known in the Army as the 90–90–90

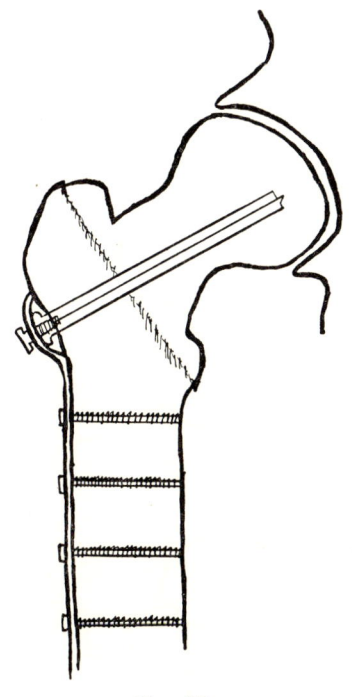

Fig. 80.

position, *i.e.*, 90 degrees flexion at hip, knee and ankle. Russell traction has proved satisfactory in certain cases. Immobilization in a plaster spica is not normally successful as shortening and angulation tend to recur. Open reduction with adequate internal fixation is frequently the treatment of choice where organization, equipment and personnel make such a procedure advisable. If traction is used, it must be maintained from eight to ten weeks. Protection by means of a well-fitting caliper brace for three to four months is a wise precaution as the callus remains soft for some time and angulation may occur.

Time of Immobilization.—If traction is used it should be maintained at least eight weeks, with brace protection for six months.

Prognosis.—This is good as far as eventual union and function are concerned, fair as regards anatomy.

Summary.—

Infrequent injuries, produced by serious accidents.

Skeletal traction usually the best form of treatment.

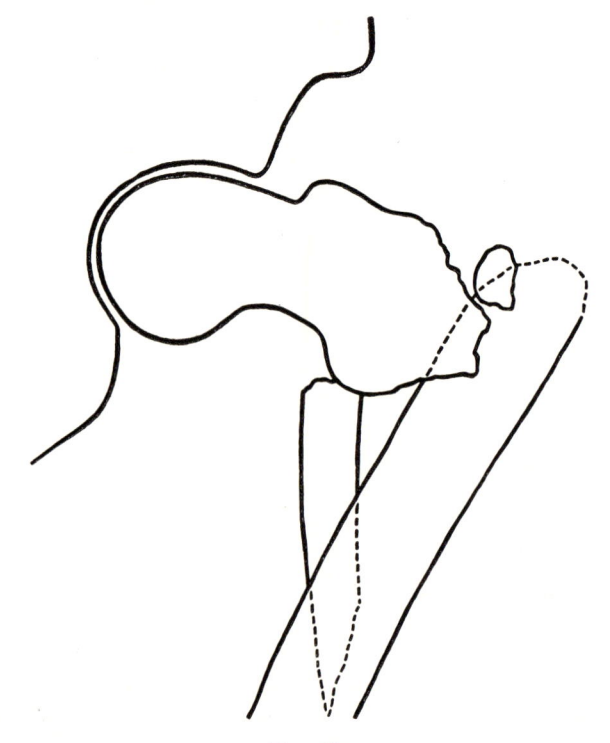

Fig. 81.

Injuries to the Hip Joint

Bony healing with mass of soft callus the usual occurrence.

Separation of the Upper Femoral Epiphysis.—*Occurrence.*—This condition is usually seen in children between the ages of ten and sixteen, frequently in the fat boy or Frölich syndrome group. It may be initiated by a very mild injury.

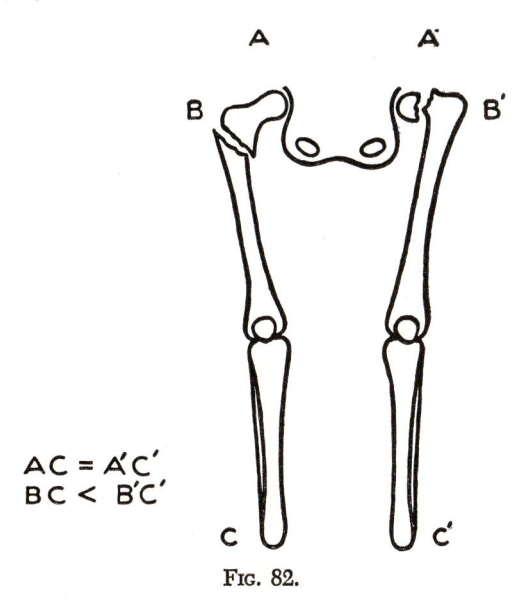

$AC = A'C'$
$BC < B'C'$

FIG. 82.

Displacement.—The head slips backward and down with the neck riding high and externally rotated.

Diagnosis.—Pain in hip or knee accompanied by a slight limp in an overweight youngster of twelve or fourteen, without serious injury, should suggest a slipped upper femoral epiphysis. If internal rotation is limited and external rotation is increased the diagnosis is strengthened. Pain in the knee may be the only presenting symptom. X-ray studies in both antero-posterior and lateral views are essential.

Pathology.—These injuries may be entirely due to trauma. On the other hand, in most cases trauma plays a minor rôle and the underlying factors are thought to be infectious, circulatory, or endocrine. Only those separations which are of traumatic origin fall within the scope of this manual.

Treatment.—Reduction can usually be accomplished if the patient is seen early enough. Gentle manipulation as for fractured femoral neck, or prolonged traction will reduce the displacement. Following reduction the epiphysis should be fused by operative means, preferably by a Smith-Petersen nail inserted through a lateral incision. Late results of cases treated by any other method are generally discouraging because of delayed changes in the femoral head.

Time of Immobilization.—For cases not operated upon, at least eight weeks in plaster or traction followed by freedom from weight-bearing for at least one year.

Prognosis.—The outlook for entirely free and painless hip motion is not favorable in many cases, as late growth disturbances and changes in the head may result.

Summary.—

- Rarely caused by trauma alone.
- Underlying condition involving the epiphysis still under discussion.
- Reduction by manipulation or traction with fixation by a Smith-Petersen nail.
- Prognosis uncertain because of late changes in the femoral head.

DISLOCATIONS AT THE HIP

Posterior Dislocations.—*Occurrence.*—These injuries are usually caused by a violent force directed proximally against the flexed knee. They are seen as the result of motor accidents, particularly jeeps, when the passenger's knee is driven violently against the dashboard.

Displacement.—The head of the femur lies behind the acetabulum with the shaft adducted and flexed.

Injuries to the Hip Joint

Diagnosis.—The deformity presented by this lesion is characteristic. The patient lies with the injured thigh flexed, adducted and internally rotated. The femoral head can usually be palpated posteriorly. Signs and symptoms of pressure on the sciatic nerve may be present.

Pathology.—Damage to the capsular structures of the hip joint is extensive and the ligamentum teres is inevitably torn across. There may be an associated fracture of the acetabular rim or, less frequently, a fracture of the femoral head. Damage to the sciatic nerve may occur.

Treatment.—Reduction as soon after injury as possible is essential. With the patient under an anesthetic, traction is exerted in the line of the flexed thigh, and by gentle rotation the head is slipped back into the acetabulum. The patient may be placed prone on a table with the thighs extending over the edge and traction exerted downward on the flexed knee. All maneuvers should be performed gently to avoid injury to the sciatic nerve. If there is a fracture of the acetabulum, closed reduction may be impossible and open reduction may be necessary. The after-care consists of balanced suspension of the limb with skin traction of about ten pounds for muscle relaxation, and early active motion within pain limits. Weight-bearing should not be permitted for several months because of the danger of aseptic necrosis of the femoral head.

Some authorities feel that patients with uncomplicated dislocations may be permitted to bear weight in four or five weeks if repeated x-rays are taken at three-month intervals to check the condition of the femoral head. Any evidence of aseptic necrosis should mean immediate non-weight-bearing.

Time of Immobilization.—Bed-rest for about two weeks followed by crutch walking without weight-bearing for at least another month, in some opinions; six months.

Prognosis.—This should be in most instances guarded because of danger of late changes in the hip.

Summary.—
  Infrequent injury caused by violent trauma.
  Manipulative reduction followed by suspension for four weeks.
  No weight-bearing from one to six months.
  Prognosis guarded because of the possibility of late changes in the femoral head and of traumatic arthritis.

Anterior Dislocations.—These are more unusual than the posterior dislocations. They are caused by a marked abduction force which pries the head out of the acetabulum anteriorly. The deformity is the opposite to the one previously described. The lower extremity is widely abducted and moderately flexed. The head of the femur can be felt in the groin. Traction in the axis of deformity and rotation will effect reduction. The subsequent treatment is the same as that outlined for the posterior dislocations.

Central Dislocations.—A violent force directed against the outer side of the thigh may drive the femoral head through the acetabulum into the pelvis. Reduction by manipulation with the use of the maneuvers used in a Whitman reduction of a femoral neck fracture may be attempted, but these injuries are frequently difficult to reduce and a continuous outward and downward pull most be exerted. This can be done by means of a Steinman pin inserted from before backward through the greater trochanter or by a screw projecting outward from the trochanter. Traction must be maintained, after the femoral head has been pulled out into normal position, until the acetabular fragments have consolidated. Active motion of the hip should be instituted as soon as possible but weight-bearing delayed for four to six months.

Chapter 18

Fractures of the Shaft of the Femur

Occurrence.—These injuries are normally the result of severe violence and occur most frequently, therefore, in active adults or in children.

Displacement.—The fracturing force is responsible for the initial position of the broken bone ends but because of the great strength of the thigh muscles the displacement is influenced by muscle pull. Overriding of the fragments is a common finding. In fractures of the upper third of the shaft, the proximal fragment is flexed by the iliopsoas (if the lesser trochanter remains attached) and abducted and externally rotated by the muscles inserted in the trochanteric region. The distal fragment is adducted by the unopposed pull of the adductors.

Diagnosis.—Because of the frequent presence of deformity the diagnosis is usually easy. X-ray films in two planes must be taken for confirmation and to ascertain the type of fracture, *i.e.*, transverse, oblique, or comminuted.

Pathology.—Because of the severity of the injury some degree of shock is almost invariably present in adults, though not usually in children. Soft tissue damage is usually extensive with tearing of the vastus intermedius and internal hemorrhage. The hematocrit readings in adults with closed femoral fractures are apt to be surprisingly low. If there is gross displacement of the fragments interposition of muscle tissue may occur.

Treatment.—In children five years old or less suspension of both lower extremities at right angles to the bed is a simple and satisfactory method of treatment (Bryant's suspension). Weight is applied by adhesive strips to the leg just sufficient to lift the buttock from the mattress (Fig.

174   Fractures of the Shaft of the Femur

83). This position is apparently perfectly comfortable for the baby, simplifies nursing care, and holds the fracture in adequate position. The adhesive strips of whatever material should be frequently checked for undue pressure, skin irritation or circulatory embarrassment. It should be main-

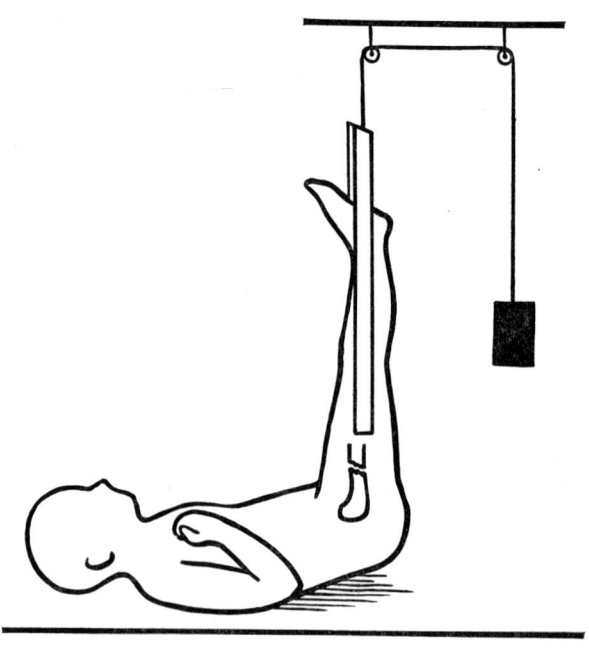

Fig. 83.

tained until there is evidence of adequate healing both clinically and by x-ray examination, usually in four weeks. The baby should not be allowed to walk for a total of about eight weeks. Immobilization of the extremity in a plaster spica with the thigh flexed and abducted in a "frog" position is another method, and satisfactory if the plaster can be kept dry.

Fractures of the femur in older children can be well treated by some form of traction suspension, preferably by

Fractures of the Shaft of the Femur

adhesive strips. Russell traction is a satisfactory method in most cases. If skeletal traction is used it is wiser to insert the pin or wire through the tibial tubercle than in the lower femoral shaft, as in the latter position the wire might cut into the epiphyseal cartilage.

In transverse fractures reduction by manipulation can frequently be done and the extremity immobilized in a plaster-of-Paris spica. Overriding of a centimeter in young children should be allowed to remain, as the inevitable overgrowth will correct the shortening. Open reduction is definitely contraindicated in children unless there is definite evidence of major circulatory damage or massive soft tissue interposition. End to end apposition of the fragments is not only not necessary but not wise.

In adults some form of traction to regain length is almost always essential. Skeletal traction, by means of a pin or a wire through the supracondylar region of the femur or through the tibial tuberosity, is the most efficient. Adequate weight should be applied to overcome the muscle spasm and regain position within the first twenty-four hours. It should then be reduced to just enough to maintain the length. Overpull should be avoided or corrected very early because of the danger of delayed or non-union. Manipulation under an anesthetic can be performed while the extremity is still in traction, to engage the fragments and correct lateral displacement. Traction should be maintained from eight to twelve weeks until there is clinical evidence of union.

Russell or Australian traction can be used for fractures of the upper and middle thirds of the femoral shaft. Its principle is based on a double pulley action (Fig. 84). It was of great value in wounds involving the upper thigh and buttock (in World War II) where it was impossible to use a Thomas splint. Reduction and fixation of fractures of the femoral shafts by double pins inserted above and below the fracture and held by an external bar is a recognized form of treatment. The Roger Anderson, Haynes and Stader appar-

176 Fractures of the Shaft of the Femur

atus are examples of this method which is particularly applicable in badly comminuted fractures.

Open reduction with rigid internal fixation is frequently the treatment of choice in adults, as it permits early active motion of the adjacent joints. Intramedullary nails, plates

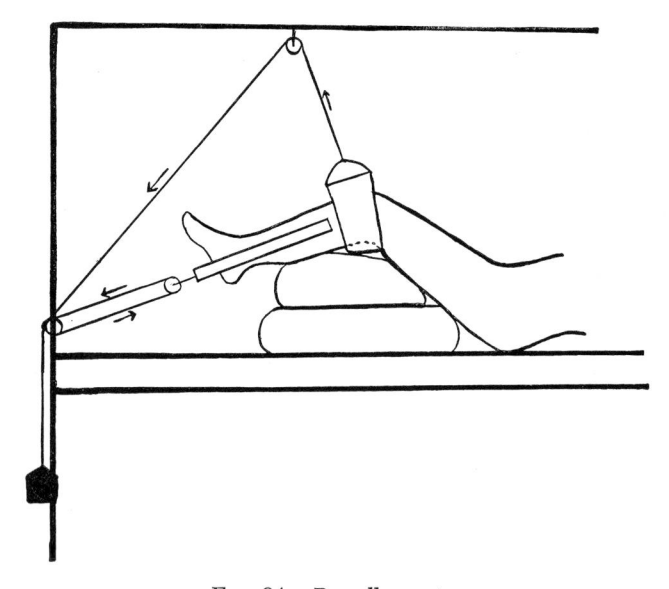

Fig. 84.—Russell traction.

and screws, or multiple screws may be employed. If adequate stabilization of the fracture has been obtained external plaster casings or spicas are unnecessary and should not be used.

A protective caliper brace is frequently advisable when closed methods of treatment have been used. It should be worn when weight-bearing is permitted for from four to six months, or until x-ray plates demonstrate firm union.

Time of Immobilization.—In children about eight weeks; in adults twelve weeks or longer.

Fractures of the Shaft of the Femur 177

Prognosis.—The prognosis should in most cases be excellent if length and axes have been restored to normal.

Summary.—

A frequent injury in children and young adults.

Bryant's suspension excellent in young children.

Manipulation and plaster-of-Paris immobilization in older children; operation usually not necessary.

Skeletal traction or open reduction with internal fixation in adults.

Interposition of soft parts a frequent complication.

Prognosis good for union and for function if length and axes are maintained.

Chapter 19

Injuries at the Knee Joint

FRACTURES OF THE LOWER EXTREMITY OF THE FEMUR

Supracondylar Fractures.—*Occurrence.*—These injuries are usually due to violent trauma and occur in active adult life. They were seen in large numbers in World War II as a result of enemy action and of jeep accidents.

Displacement.—Although this depends primarily on the fracturing force, the characteristic displacement of the distal fragment is posterior due to the action of the gastrocnemius muscle (Fig. 85).

Diagnosis.—Swelling may obscure the bony landmarks but frequently the lower end of the upper fragment can be palpated. X-ray examination is essential for details of the injury.

Pathology.—Soft part damage is always extensive and occasionally the circulation of the leg may be compromised by extensive internal hemorrhage. Direct injury to the large blood-vessels may be caused by the distal fragment.

Treatment.—Immediate reduction is essential. Manual reduction alone is seldom successful unless the patient is seen immediately after injury. Skeletal traction by means of pin or wire through the upper end of the tibia with the knee flexed is a satisfactory method and may be coupled with direct manipulation. If the reduction is satisfactory, a plaster spica can be applied incorporating the pin, or continuous pull can be maintained by some form of traction suspension. A second pin through the distal fragment exerting anterior pull may be necessary in some cases to correct the deformity. If the blood supply to the limb has

Injuries to the Knee Joint

been damaged immediate operation is indicated and internal fixaton of the fragments may be employed. In certain cases, where the obliquity and height of the fracture line permits, internal fixation may be the method of choice. Anatomical alignment must be restored, if possible, because

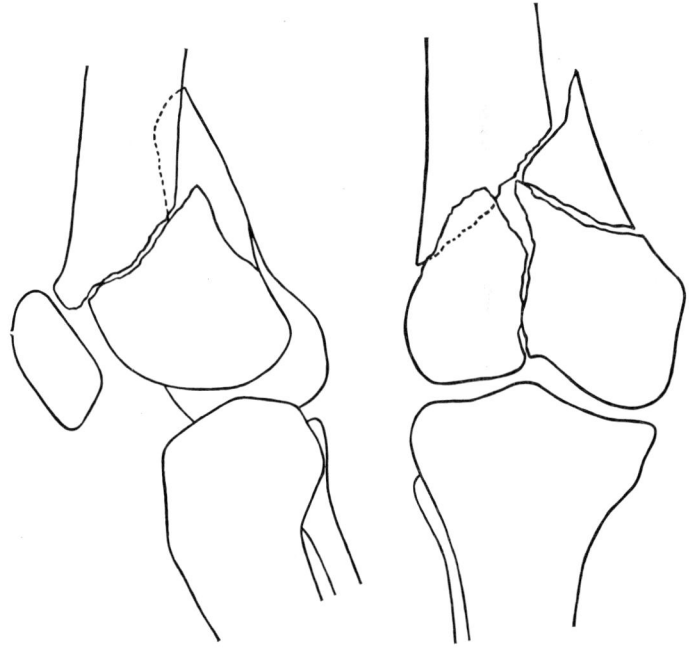

FIG. 85.

any residual deformity will result in a change in the lower articular surface of the femur and a resultant disability in the knee-joint.

Active muscle contractions should be encouraged from the onset of treatment, whether immobilization or continuous traction be used. Active motion should be started at from six to eight weeks but unprotected weight-bearing should not be permitted for about twelve weeks after injury.

Injuries to the Knee Joint

If rigid internal fixation has been obtained, active exercises can be instituted much earlier.

Time of Immobilization.—From six to eight weeks in plaster or continuous traction, about three months before full weight-bearing is permitted.

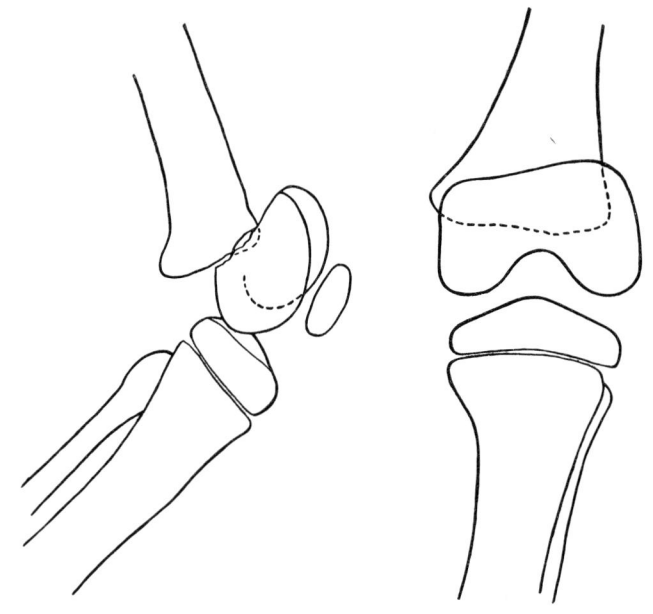

Fig. 86.

Prognosis.—Bony union is the rule and if anatomical restoration has been obtained the ultimate function should be good. Full knee motion may be delayed.

Summary.—

    Caused by violent trauma.

    Posterior displacement of distal fragment characteristic.

    Treated by pin traction through flexed knee, operation occasionally necessary.

    Immobilization for from six to eight weeks with freedom from weight-bearing for three months.

Injuries to the Knee Joint

Separation of the Lower Femoral Epiphysis.—*Occurrence.*—These fractures are seen in children, usually between the ages of eight and fourteen years, though they may occur at any age up to the time of closure of the epiphyseal line. They are the result of severe accidents.

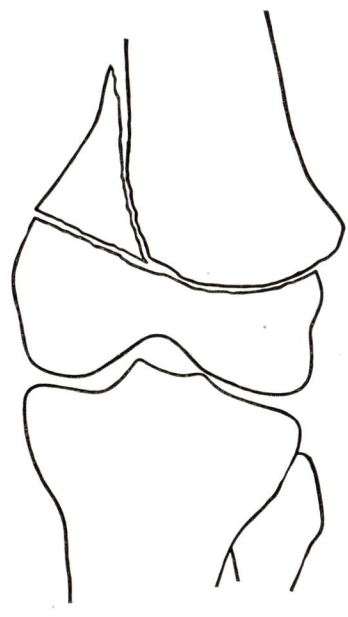

FIG. 87.

Displacment.—The epiphysis may be displaced forward or backward, depending on the fracturing force (Fig. 86). A lateral or a medial shift may also occur and rotation of the distal fragment is occasionally seen. Frequently the epiphysis takes with it a wedge-shaped fragment of the diaphysis (Fig. 87).

Diagnosis.—Symptoms and signs of fracture at the lower extremity of a femur of a child should strongly suggest the diagnosis. X-ray examination is essential.

Injuries to the Knee Joint

Pathology.—Because of the severity of the injury there is usually considerable soft part damage. Occasionally the displacement is so marked that the popliteal vessels and nerves are injured.

Treatment.—Reduction under anesthesia can usually be satisfactorily accomplished if the patient is seen early. Relaxation of the gastrocnemius by flexion of the knee helps in the manipulation. After the epiphysis has been replaced it can be held in position by molded splints or a circular plaster casing with the knee semi-flexed. If there is evidence of circulatory embarrassment immediate operation may be necessary. Immobilization should be maintained for about four weeks.

Time of Immobilization.—Usually four weeks.

Prognosis.—There is normally complete return of function in about six months. Growth disturbances are not infrequent however, and may take place on one side of the epiphyseal cartilage only, resulting in marked deformity.

Summary.—

  Injury caused by severe trauma.

  Deformity frequently marked.

  Treatment, manipulative reduction followed by immobilization for four weeks. Surgical intervention necessary in rare cases.

  Prognosis guarded because of danger of growth disturbance.

FRACTURES OF THE PATELLA

Occurrence.—These are of fairly frequent occurrence and may be caused either by direct or by indirect violence.

Displacement.—If the blow is direct the fracture is apt to be stellate or fragmented and not displaced (Fig. 88). If, however, indirect violence, either alone or coupled with direct violence, is the causative factor there is usually tearing of the aponeurotic expansion of the quadriceps (Fig. 89). Contraction of that muscle pulls the proximal frag-

Injuries to the Knee Joint

ment upward frequently for a distance of some centimeters.

Diagnosis.—Because of the superficial position of the patella the deformity is easily palpated in most instances. Occasionally the soft part damage is so great that the bony outline cannot be felt. X-ray films taken not only in the antero-posterior and lateral planes but also, in obscure cases,

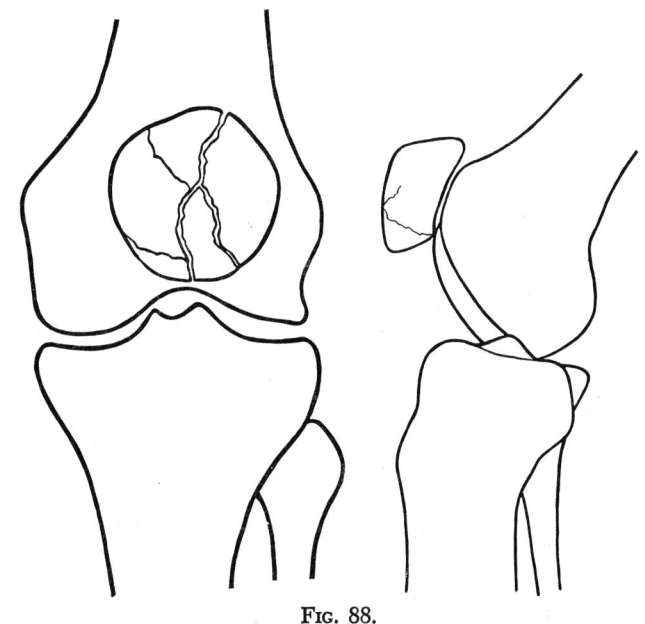

Fig. 88.

from above downward through the flexed knee will give the diagnosis.

Pathology.—The most important consideration in these injuries is the integrity of the soft parts. The patella is actually a sesamoid bone in the quadriceps tendon and may be crushed by a direct blow without tearing the surrounding soft tissue. If such be the case the problem is much simplified. On the other hand if the aponeurosis is torn opening the joint and separating the bony fragments, the situation is more complicated.

Injuries to the Knee Joint

Treatment.—When there has been no separation of the fragments aspiration of the hemarthrosis will make the patient much more comfortable and enable him to move his knee more easily. Frequently no immobilization other than a pressure bandage is necessary, and weight-bearing may be allowed from the onset. If there is separation of the

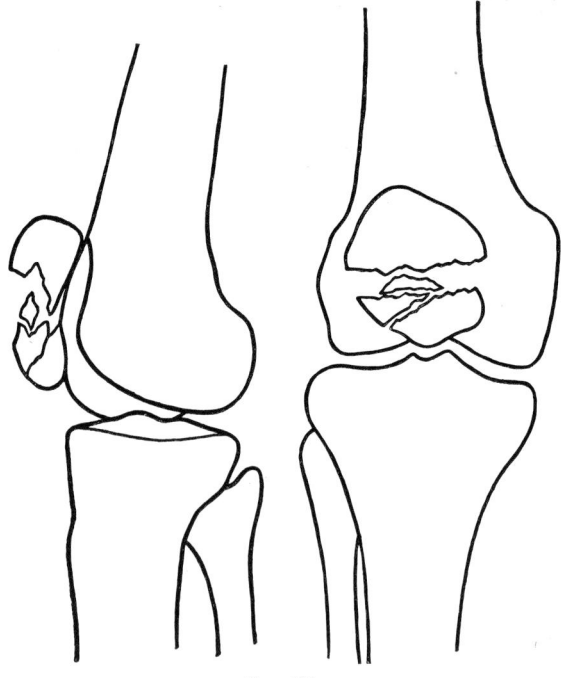

Fig. 89.

fragments, the best form of treatment is that of open reduction and fixation of the fragments by some means, fascia, wire, silk, etc., coupled with a careful repair of the aponeurosis and capsule. If the repair is sufficiently firm, guarded active motion may be begun within a week, but unprotected weight-bearing should not be allowed for from four to six weeks. Complete excision of the patella is not advised

Injuries to the Knee Joint

unless the bone is completely shattered. Frequently there is a fairly large segment of the proximal portion of the patella that is intact and should be left with removal of the smaller distal fragments (Fig. 89). In all cases repair of the aponeurosis is essential. Active contraction of the quadriceps should be initiated as soon as possible after operation. If for some reason operation is impossible, the separate fragments may be pulled together to some extent by strips of adhesive on the skin and the extremity then immobilized in extension in circular plaster for from four to six weeks. This is, however, a very poor second best.

Time of Immobilization.—Two or three weeks in fractures without separation. Protection for four weeks after operation but early guarded motion.

Prognosis.—If the articular surface heals smoothly the patient should have a satisfactorily functioning knee. Irregularities on the articular surface may cause pain on certain motions. As a rule the prognosis is good.

Summary.—

Caused by direct or indirect violence.

Undisplaced fractures: treatment by pressure bandage or splint for two weeks followed by active motion.

Displaced fracture: treatment by open reduction, internal fixation and repair of aponeurosis; guarded weight-bearing in four weeks.

Prognosis usually good.

FRACTURES OF THE UPPER EXTREMITY OF THE TIBIA

Occurrence.—These injuries are increasing with the frequency of automobile accidents. Many of them are caused by a blow from a car bumper.

Displacement.—The fracture line may be completely across the upper end of the tibia, it may be T- or Y-shaped, or it may involve one condyle only. The most frequent site of injury is the lateral condyle, the cause a blow on the outer aspect of the knee joint with forceful abduction of the leg on the thigh (Fig. 90). The condyle is frequently displaced downward, sometimes in one piece, sometimes crushed in many pieces. If the blow is on the medial aspect of the knee, forced adduction may cause a depression of the medial condyle.

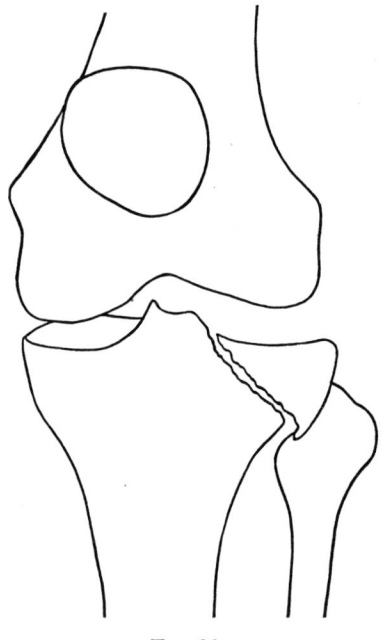

Fig. 90.

Diagnosis.—There may be definite change in the axis of the leg on the thigh, depending on the amount of depression of the condyle. There is frequently considerable swelling, with a marked hemarthrosis if the capsule of the joint remains intact. Instability of the knee joint with increase in ab- or adduction depending on the site of injury is evidence of a torn collateral ligament. If there is acute tenderness on the side opposite to that of the torn ligament, that is, if in a

Injuries to the Knee Joint

patient whose leg can be abnormally abducted on the thigh there is tenderness over the lateral tibial condyle, it is indicative of a fracture of the condyle as well as a tear of the medial collateral ligament. Occasionally a tear of the ligament only may result from such an injury, in which case with a blow on the outer side of the knee all the signs and symptoms will be referred to the medial side. X-ray pictures are essential for the diagnosis.

Pathology.—As always with a fracture into a joint, one of the presenting symptoms is that of blood in the joint accumulating gradually in the first hours after the accident. Tearing of the collateral ligament, as has been mentioned, is a frequent complication. The semilunar cartilages may also be torn or detached at the time of injury. Because of the character of the bone involved in the fracture the deformity may gradually increase if too early weight-bearing is allowed; the cancellous bone may crush down if the weight of the body is applied before the healing process is firm. If there is also a fracture of the fibular neck, damage to the peroneal nerve may occur either at the time of injury or later from pressure by the callus.

Treatment.—In cases where the displacement is negligible, aspiration of the joint followed by elevation and immobilization for two or three days is the initial treatment. Active motion without weight-bearing should be begun as soon as the swelling and tenderness have subsided. This can be most easily accomplished in a suspension apparatus with a hinged footpiece and skin traction on the lower leg of 2 or 3 pounds' weight to pull the joint surfaces apart. This should be continued for two or three weeks, after which the patient should be allowed up and permitted to walk with crutches without bearing weight on the affected leg. If the portion of the condyle involved in the fracture is small, weight-bearing may be begun somewhat sooner. If it involves a considerable portion of the articular surface, however, even with no initial displacement of the fragment, weight-bearing should not be permitted until after twelve weeks from the time of injury. In cases with gross displacement open reduction is the method of choice. If the fragment is large it can frequently be held in position by screws or wires. Sometimes the condyle can be pushed up into position and held by a bone graft beneath it. Attempts at closed reduction are usually unsuccessful, and the immobilization necessary to maintain any correction will result in a stiffened joint. Occasionally the displacement may be corrected by traction, either skin or skeletal, in either abduction or adduction, depending on the deformity, with swathes on the apparatus to maintain side pull.

Period of Immobilization.—No weight-bearing for twelve weeks.

Prognosis.—If there has been little deformity so that active motion can be maintained almost from the beginning, the prognosis should be good. If immobilization is necessary there may be limitation of the full range of motion. Residual deformity may result in pain and limitation of function.

Summary.—

Frequent injury from automobile bumpers.

Lateral condyle usually depressed and may be associated with tearing of medial collateral ligament.

If undisplaced, aspiration and early active motion without weight-bearing.

If displaced, open reduction with internal fixation.

No weight-bearing for twelve weeks unless insignificant portion of articular surface involved.

Prognosis for function guarded.

Fractures of the Tibial Spine.—These injuries may occur from indirect violence and are frequently due to the pull of the crucial ligaments. If there is little or no displacement, immobilization of the knee in extension for three or four weeks is all that is necessary. If there is great displacement, open reduction must be done with fixation of the fragment, or, if that is not possible, with its removal.

Chapter 20

Fractures of the Shafts of the Tibia and Fibula

Occurrence.—These injuries are due either to direct or indirect violence and usually occur in children and young adults leading an active and strenuous existence.

Displacement.—If the blow is direct the fracture line is usually transverse with a triangular fragment frequently split off on the side opposite to that which received the blow (Fig. 91). Both bones are broken at the same level. If the violence is indirect the fracture line is spiral or oblique with the fibular break usually higher than that of the tibia (Fig. 92). The initial displacement is caused by the fracturing force and overriding by muscular action or by the patient's attempts to stand immediately after the accident.

Diagnosis.—In cases where there is any displacement the diagnosis is obvious. Deformity, crepitus and false point of motion are all present. Where there is no displacement, especially in the injuries of young children where the fracture may be subperiosteal, a line of bony tenderness, indirect tenderness, and a refusal to use the extremity on the part of the youngster should suggest the diagnosis. X-ray films in two planes should be taken to include the entire length of the tibia as second fracture lines may be otherwise missed.

Pathology.—These are injuries of violence and in most cases there is apt to be extensive soft part damage with considerable bleeding within the tissues. The skin may be avulsed or lifted up from the underlying soft parts by hemorrhage, as in cases where a wheel passes over the leg. Open fractures are frequently seen. Circulatory embarrass-

Fractures of Shaft of Tibia and Fibula

ment due to the tense swelling of the calf may occur. Volkmann's paralysis of the lower extremity has been reported, though less frequently than in the upper extremity. Delayed or non-union is a not infrequent result of fractures of the tibial shaft.

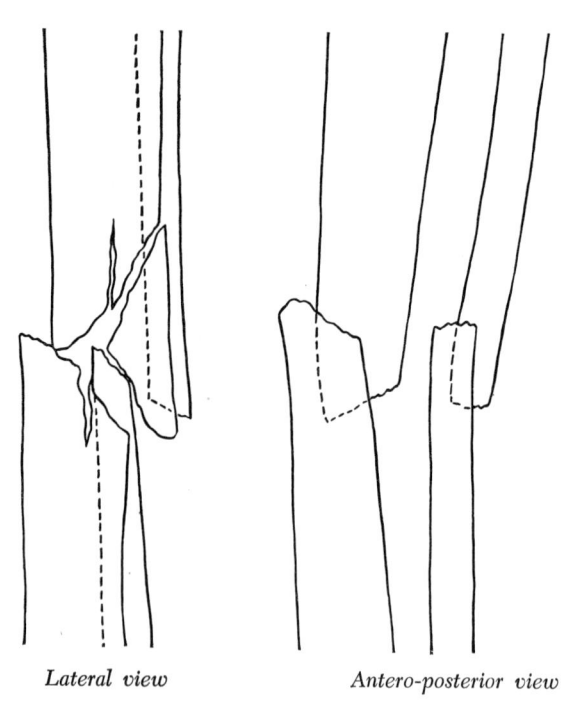

Lateral view   *Antero-posterior view*

Fig. 91.

Treatment.—Three methods of treatment are in use at the present time for these injuries depending on the kind of fracture and the desires of the surgeon. In most fractures in children, in undisplaced fractures in adults and in transverse fractures that can be locked by manipulation, closed reduction followed by immobilization in posterior molded and sugar tongs splints or circular plaster from toes to groin

Fractures of Shaft of Tibia and Fibula

is satisfactory. The knee must be flexed to 135 degrees. In spiral fractures, in those which tend to slip after reduction, and in those with comminution, immobilization by plaster alone is usually not adequate. Traction is necessary for maintenance of position and may be supplied by pins or wires incorporated in the plaster casing after reduction has

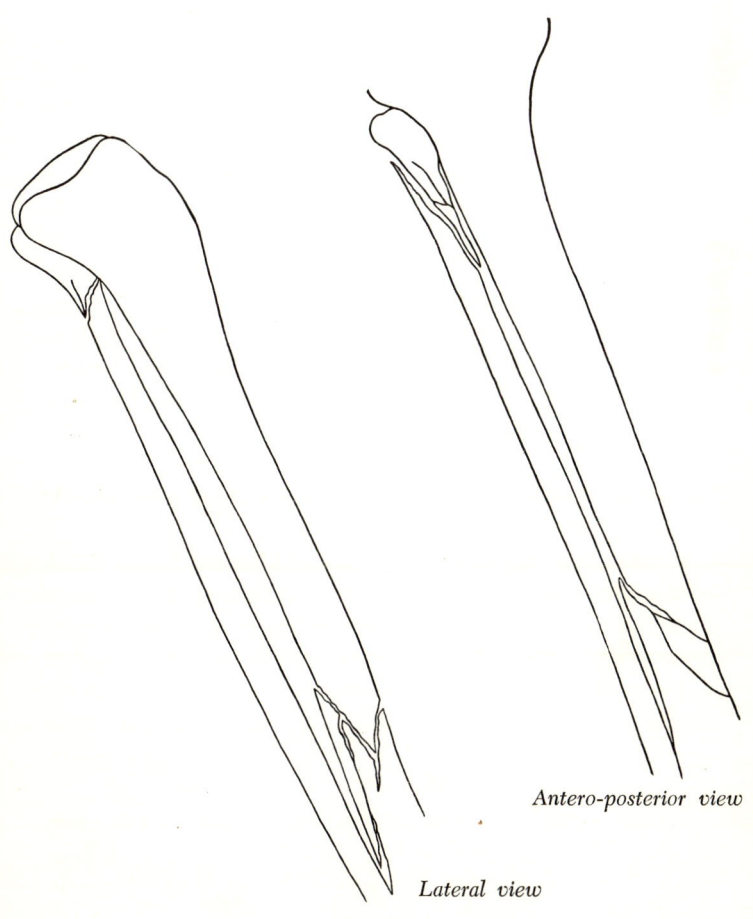

Antero-posterior view

Lateral view

Fig. 92.

Fractures of Shaft of Tibia and Fibula

been obtained or by various pin and external splint techniques like the Roger Anderson, the Stader or the Haynes apparatus. In any of these methods, great care must be taken to avoid overpull. After length has been obtained, the fragments should be held pressed together by the apparatus. In certain instances, where normal length and correct weight-bearing axis cannot be obtained or maintained by other methods, open reduction becomes a necessity. Because of the early exercise of function afforded by open reduction with rigid internal fixation, it is the method of choice in those institutions where the organization for such a procedure is adequate.

Whichever method is used, elevation of the extremity is necessary in the first few days until the swelling has subsided. Union of the fracture cannot be expected before eight weeks and in many cases may be delayed considerably longer. If any form of plaster casing has been used, Unna paste stockings or elastic bandages should be applied following the removal of the plaster, as some edema of the extremity is inevitable. If rigid fixation by internal means has been obtained, active motion should be encouraged, and weight-bearing can be allowed in a brace at six weeks. If normal circulation has been restored, swelling in these cases should not be troublesome.

Fractures at the junction of the middle and lower thirds of the tibia are apt to be slow in healing and may proceed to a fibrous union. If this occurs multiple drilling, massive bone grafts, chip grafts, are methods of treatment suggested.

Time of Immobilization.—If plaster-of-Paris or one of the methods of pin traction is used, it should be maintained for from eight to ten weeks. A leg brace or a walking plaster boot may be necessary thereafter if union is delayed.

Prognosis.—This should be good in children and in many adults. It should be definitely guarded, however, in fractures of the tibia at the middle and lower third where delayed union may result.

Fractures of Shaft of Tibia and Fibula

Summary.—
   Severe direct or indirect violence the usual cause.
   Reduction and immobilization in plaster satisfactory for fractures in children and in undisplaced fractures of adults.
   Wires above and below the fracture and incorporated in the plaster casing valuable in oblique fractures.
   Open reduction occasionally necessary.
   Delayed and non-union a danger.
   Prognosis guarded.

Fractures of the Shaft of the Fibula.—These injuries are usually due to direct violence, a blow against the outer side of the leg. The displacement is negligible if the tibia is intact and the treatment is merely that of protection against further injury. A lateral splint and the use of crutches for a week or so are all that is required.

Chapter 21

Injuries at the Ankle Joint

FRACTURES OF THE MALLEOLI

Fractures of the Lateral Malleolus.—*Occurrence.*—These injuries are very common and may be due to a sudden twisting of the foot or, less frequently, to a blow on the outer side of the ankle. They usually occur in active young adults but may be seen at any age.

Displacement.—The fracture is usually caused by outward rotation of the foot resulting in a spiral or oblique fracture line. Marked displacement cannot occur without an associated tear of the internal collateral ligament or a fracture of the medial malleolus. Sudden inversion of the foot may pull off the tip of the lateral malleous but the ligament is more apt to give way, resulting in a sprain rather than a fracture.

Diagnosis.—Direct tenderness over the lateral malleolus suggests the presence of a fracture. X-ray examination is essential for confirmation, for occasionally the tenderness in a sprain may be misleading. The medial aspect of the ankle should be examined for signs of a torn ligament.

Pathology.—There is usually swelling with ecchymosis spreading down along the outside of the foot depending on the extent of the soft part damage. Injury to nerves and large blood-vessels is not usual.

Treatment.—If there has been no displacement of the fragment, adhesive strapping protection and early weight-bearing may be permitted. Extensive swelling may necessitate rest, elevation and heat for a few days before the strapping can be applied. More severe injuries, especially those requiring manipulative reduction, should be immobilized in posterior molded and sugar tongs splints to the knee until the immediate swelling has subsided, then in a walking plaster boot for from three to four weeks. Following the removal of the plaster, adhesive strapping or an ankle brace should be used.

It should be emphasized that a walking plaster, *i.e.*, a circular plaster casing fitted with a heel, a rocker, or an iron, is designed for protected weight-bearing to enable the patient to use the muscles of the injured leg. Care must be taken to see that the patient understands this and that he actually walks on the leg. Otherwise the purpose of the walking plaster is lost and prolonged stiffness of the ankle will result.

Time of Immobilization.—No immobilization may be needed in minor injuries without displacement, but protection up to six weeks is called for in the more severe ones.

Prognosis.—This should be good.

Summary.—

Frequent injury usually caused by outward rotation of the foot.

Treatment, early weight-bearing with adhesive strapping or walking plaster depending on severity.

Soft part damage important consideration.

Immobilization in severe cases four to six weeks.

Prognosis good.

Fractures of the Medial Malleolus.—*Occurrence.*—Isolated fractures of the medial malleolus are less common than those of the lateral but are occasionally seen. They are caused by abduction or adduction of the foot.

Displacement.—If the injury is that of forcible abduction there will be a transverse fracture of the malleolus. If it is that of adduction the fracture line will be oblique.

Diagnosis.—Localized tenderness over the medial malleolus is significant. X-rays are necessary for confirmation.

Pathology.—Frequently in the transverse fractures, a flap of torn periosteum is pulled into the fracture line and as a result fibrous union is not uncommon.

Injuries at the Ankle Joint

Treatment.—If there is no displacement and the soft part damage is minimal, early weight-bearing with adhesive strapping or a walking plaster for two to three weeks gives satisfactory results. If, on the other hand, there is any displacement and the fragment comprises a major portion of

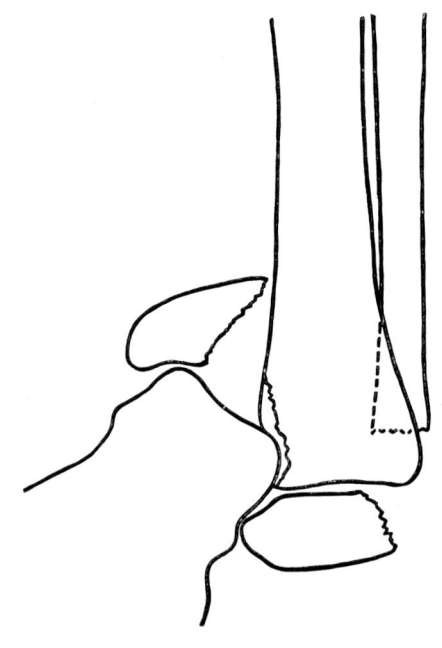

Fig. 93.

the malleolus, so that the integrity of the mortise is threatened, open reduction with fixation by a screw or peg after removal of the interposed periosteal flap is the method of choice. No immobilization is needed and early active motion should be instituted. Protected weight-bearing with adhesive strapping or ankle brace can be permitted within two weeks.

Time of Immobilization.—Two to four weeks if necessary.
Prognosis.—Fibrous union may result. If the fragment is

Injuries at the Ankle Joint

small function will be good. If the fragment is relatively large and bony union does not occur a weak and painful ankle may persist. Oblique fractures usually heal rapidly with bony union.

Summary.—

Infrequent injuries.

Interposition of periosteum not uncommon.

Open reduction with internal fixation frequently necessary.

Fibrous union qualifies prognosis.

Fractures of Both Malleoli.—*Occurrence.*—These injuries are caused by considerable violence, frequently by a fall on a twisted foot. They occur usually in people engaged in strenuous activities.

Displacement.—The foot with the malleoli may be displaced either outward or inward, depending upon the direction of the fracturing force. Displacement in these cases may be very marked (Fig. 93). Because of the pull of the calf muscles there is almost always a backward displacement as well. There may or may not be a fracture of the posterior lip of the tibia.

Diagnosis.—The ankle is a hinged joint formed by the lateral malleolus, the inferior tibio-fibular ligament, the tibial articular surface and the medial malleolus as one element and the talus as the other. The upper surface of the talus is curved convexly from before backward, which allows it to rock on the tibial surface and permits flexion and extension of the foot on the leg. Lateral, medial, or rotary motion of the talus is normally impossible because of the "mortise" shape of the joint (Fig. 94). Inversion, eversion and rotation of the foot take place in the subtalar and midtarsal joints. The malleoli are subcutaneous and easily palpable. The tip of the lateral malleolus lies distal and slightly posterior to the medial. A line dropped from the anterior-superior spine of the ilium through the patella should pass through the center of the talus. It is important for the function of the joint that the mortise be restored and the weight-bearing axis maintained.

In bi-malleolar fractures the deformity is frequently marked and the diagnosis therefore obvious. If there is no gross displacement the diagnosis is suggested by localized tenderness over both malleoli. X-ray films are necessary to show the details of the fractures.

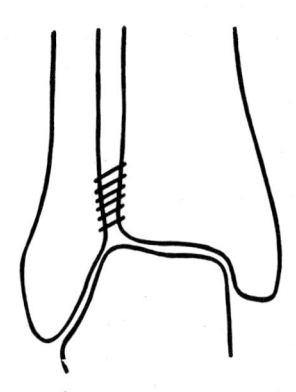

Fig. 94.

Pathology.—The foot and the malleolar fragments are usually displaced "in one piece" with the ligaments remaining intact. Occasionally the skin is stretched over the proximal fragment with subsequent necrosis. Compounding is not infrequent. Massive swelling is almost always present. Nerve and large vessel injuries are rare.

Treatment.—The earlier the reduction the easier it is. If seen within a few hours of injury, before the swelling has become marked, anatomical reduction of a marked displacement can frequently be obtained. The knee must be flexed to relax the gastrocnemius and traction exerted on the foot. The malleoli can be molded into position by direct pressure. Following reduction the ankle should be immobilized in posterior molded and sugar tongs splints carried above the knee to maintain its flexion and prevent recur-

Injuries at the Ankle Joint

rence of backward displacement. The foot should be held at right angles to the leg and the heel in very slight inversion. Marked inversion will force the talus against the fibular fragment displacing it outward. Elevation of the extremity immediately following reduction is essential to combat the inevitable swelling. Circular plaster should not be used on a fresh fracture unless it is immediately split for its full length. The splints may be replaced by a walking plaster boot after two to three weeks and the patient encouraged to walk. Frequent x-ray checks are necessary in the first few weeks to make sure that position has been maintained. All plaster can be removed at eight weeks and the patient allowed to walk with adhesive protection. The pain from a traumatic flat foot frequently seen following these injuries can be to a large measure prevented by raising the inner side of the heel of the shoe before weight-bearing is allowed.

Time of Immobilization.—Adequate splinting should be maintained for from six to eight weeks.

Prognosis.—If a satisfactory reduction has been maintained the functional result is usually good. Swelling at the end of the day may persist for months.

Summary.—

Severe violence usually causative factor.

Deformity usually marked with displacement of foot either inward or outward, and backward.

Treatment—reduction with immobilization in splints followed by walking iron for from six to eight weeks.

Prognosis is usually good.

Fractures of the Lower Third of the Fibular Shaft and the Medial Malleolus Associated With Separation of the Inferior Tibio-fibular Ligament (Pott's).—These fractures are of considerable importance, although they are not common. They are caused by a violent twist of the foot outward, frequently with rotation. The result of this force is to pull off the medial malleolus and pry the fibula outward, rupturing the inferior tibio-fibular ligament and breaking the fibula through the lower part of the shaft (Fig. 95). The foot is displaced outward, backward and upward, and the deformity may be marked. Early reduction is not difficult if the leg is kept flexed on the thigh in order to relax the gastrocnemius muscle. Traction downward overcomes the

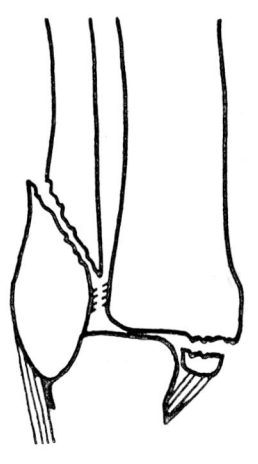

Fig. 95.

shortening. Pressure forward on the calcaneus corrects the backward displacement and the foot may then be placed in correct line with the tibia and held there by firm pressure on the malleoli to compress the widened mortise.

Following reduction, posterior molded and sugar tongs splints from the toes to as near the groin as possible should be applied while the foot is held in position and the malleoli are held pressed tightly together. The foot should be at right angles to the leg with the heel in very slight inversion and the forefoot in neutral position. Marked inversion of the foot tends to displace the fibular fragment. This position should be maintained for about four weeks with tightening of the bandages as the swelling diminishes. It is necessary to keep the knee immobilized in flexion for this period to prevent backward displacement of the foot. A walking boot should not be used in these cases because of the great danger of displacement. At four weeks the splints may be cut below the knee and after six weeks may be removed for soaks and active exercises. Weight-bearing, however, should not be allowed before ten weeks because of the risk of stretching the damaged inferior tibio-fibular ligaments. If patients with this injury are permitted to walk too soon a widened mortise and an unstable joint may thus result. A lift on the inner side of the shoe when weight-bearing is allowed will tend to prevent traumatic flat-foot, and elastic bandages will prevent excessive swelling of the lower extremity. Return to function is usually complete between six and eight months. Moderate edema of the ankle may last considerably longer than that. Because of the long period of treatment needed in these cases open reduction has been advocated, with replacement of the fragments and fixation of the fibula to the tibia by screws or a bolt. This allows the patient to be up and back at work weeks before he would be able to walk if treated by the other method.

Separation of the Epiphysis.—Injury to the epiphysis of either tibia or fibula may occur with or without displacement. If there is displacement, reduction must be done. The ankle is then immobilized, either in posterior molded and sugar tongs splints or in a walking boot, for about six weeks. If there is no displacement, protection by splints or boot should be maintained until all tenderness has disappeared. In most instances the prognosis is good, but the danger of growth disturbance should be remembered even in those cases where there has been no gross displacement.

FRACTURES OF THE LOWER EXTREMITY OF THE TIBIA

Complicated Fracture of the Lower Extremity of the Tibia.—Occasionally a comminuted fracture of the tibia with multiple fracture lines into the joint may be caused by a fall from a height. This type of injury is frequently very difficult to reduce. A wire through the calcaneus and one through the tibial shaft may be used to pull the fragments into position. The wires may be incorporated in a plaster boot and the patient allowed up after the danger of further swelling has passed. Frequently, however, traction will not influence some of the fragments and open reduction is indicated. The prognosis should be guarded because of the possibility of the development of traumatic arthritis and pain on weight-bearing.

DISLOCATIONS AT THE ANKLE JOINT

Pure dislocations are extremely rare. They are almost invariably associated with a fracture or with a rupture of the inferior tibio-fibular ligament. Reduction by manipulation followed by immobilization, as previously described, is the method of treatment.

Chapter 22

Injuries to the Foot

FRACTURES OF THE TARSUS

Fractures of the Talus.—*Occurrence.*—These injuries occur usually in active adults and are most frequently due to severe trauma. Though relatively uncommon in civilian life they were seen in large numbers in World War II as a result of jeep accidents, mine explosions and airplane crashes.

Displacement.—The fracture may be insignificant, an avulsion caused by the pull of a ligament; it may be severe, a break through the neck caused by forced hyperflexion (Fig. 96), or a crush due to a force exerted upward from below.

Diagnosis.—Tenderness just below the level of the distal tibial articular surface is suggestive but x-rays are essential.

Pathology.—If there is gross displacement, with dislocation of the body of the bone, there is almost inevitably damage to the blood supply with the threat of impending aseptic necrosis.

Treatment.—If the fracture is insignificant and due to a ligamentous pull the treatment should be directed to the soft part pathology. If, however, the fracture is severe and the displacement marked, immediate reduction by manipulation in marked plantar flexion should be attempted. Skeletal traction may be necessary. Open reduction may have to be resorted to if closed methods fail. Removal of the bone should not be done if it can possibly be avoided as the resulting foot is deformed and painful. Following reduction, immobilization in a plaster boot with the foot in equinus should be maintained for about two weeks. The foot should then be brought up to the neutral position and immobilized in plaster for another four weeks. Following the removal of the plaster, non-weight-bearing exercises should be instituted to restore the mobility and musculature

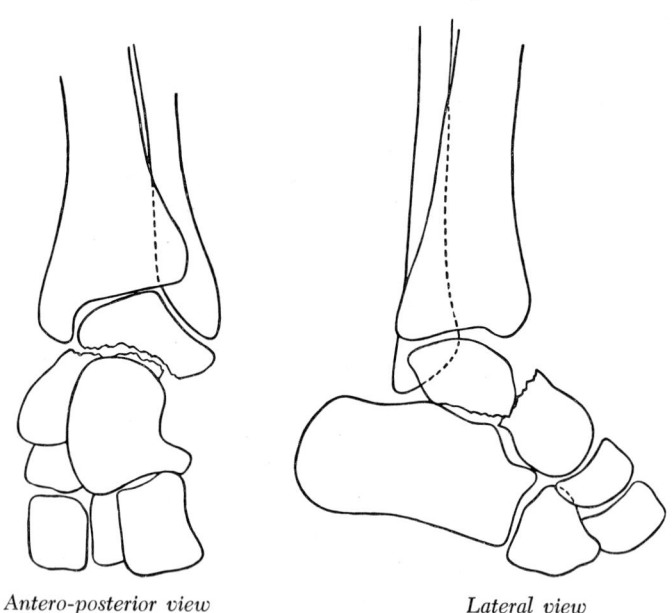

Antero-posterior view *Lateral view*
Fig. 96.—Fracture of the talus.

of leg and foot, but weight-bearing should not be started for from eight to ten weeks.

Time of Immobilization.—The plaster boot should be maintained for six weeks but unprotected weight-bearing not started for eight to ten weeks.

Prognosis.—Because of the danger of aseptic necrosis and traumatic arthritis the prognosis should be guarded.

Summary.—

An uncommon injury caused by forced dorsi-flexion or by upward force.

Reduction urgent, by manipulation in plantar flexion.

Injuries to the Foot

Immobilization in plaster boot six weeks.
No weight-bearing for at least eight weeks.
Prognosis guarded.

Fractures of the Calcaneus.—*Occurrence.*—These are the most frequent fractures of the tarsus and are usually caused by a fall from a height, the patient landing on the heels. They were frequently seen in World War II as a result of mine and torpedo explosions with the fracturing force directed upward against the feet of men in trucks or on the decks of ships. Associated compression fracture of the vertebral bodies should always be considered.

Displacement.—The postero-superior angle of the bone may be pulled off by the Achilles tendon or broken by direct violence and then displaced upward by the contraction of the calf muscles. On the other hand there may be a complete fracture through the body of the bone or a comminution with widening of the transverse diameter and a flattening of the superior surface.

Pathology.—Swelling is often marked for some days after injury. Healing will occur because of adequate blood supply but an irregularity of the superior articular surface of the calcaneus may persist, resulting in traumatic arthritis of the subtalar joint and a painful foot.

Treatment.—If the postero-superior angle has been pulled or knocked off it may be held in place by immobilizing the foot in plantar flexion and the knee flexed. The best procedure, however, is open reduction with some form of internal fixation and early active motion. If the fracture is comminuted with disturbance of the articular surface, or if there is upward tilt of a large posterior fragment, the deformity may be overcome by the distraction pull of two wires or pins, one through the posterior fragment and one through the tibia (Fig. 97). The knee must be flexed to relax the pull of the gastrocnemius. The broadening of the heel due to the crushing of the bone can be corrected either by direct manual pressure or, better, by a well-padded vise

Injuries to the Foot

or compression clamp. Because of the intense swelling in many of these cases it may be wise to defer reduction for twenty-four or forty-eight hours while attempts are made to reduce the swelling by pressure bandages, elevation and physical therapy. Following reduction the pins or wires

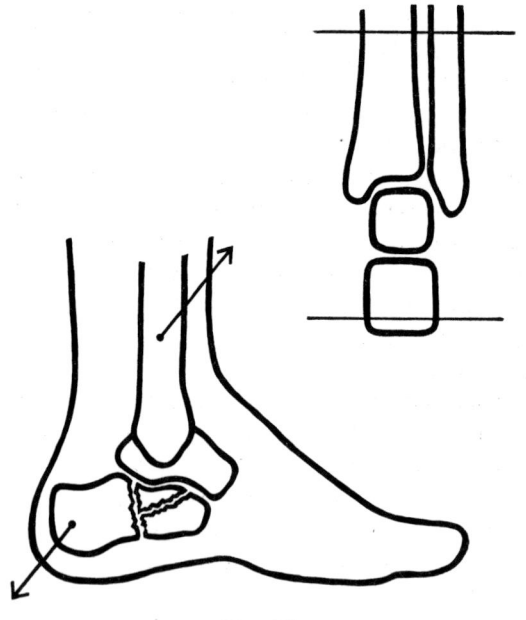

Fig. 97.

should be incorporated in a plaster boot for eight weeks. Because of the unsatisfactory results usually obtained by the closed reduction methods, early operative interference has been advised by some authorities. Others have recommended immediate closed reduction with splint protection for about a week, followed by active motion of the foot and ankle with hot soaks and elevation. This method prevents fibrosis of the intrinsic muscles of the foot and adhesions in the subtalar joint. If there is little or no displacement of the fracture, immobilization is not indicated but every attempt should be made to restore the normal physiology of the foot by non-weight-bearing exercises. In no case should weight-bearing be permitted before eight weeks, in some cases twelve weeks and then only in a specially built shoe with a prolonged counter and a hollowed heel.

Time of Immobilization.—Preferably no immobilization, but no weight-bearing for ten or twelve weeks.

Prognosis.—In severe injuries this should be guarded as painful walking due to traumatic arthritis of the subtalar joint may result.

Summary.—

Causative factor a fall from a height.

Crushing injury with widening of the bone and upward angulation of the posterior portion.

Reduction by wire pull and manipulation.

Prognosis guarded.

Other Fractures of the Tarsus.—These are of infrequent occurrence and relatively little importance. Soft part damage should receive the first consideration.

FRACTURES OF THE METATARSALS

These injuries are frequently caused by direct violence, usually of the crushing type, and are characterized by considerable soft tissue damage. The displacement is usually due to the direction of the fracturing force. Reduction of the displacement can frequently be accomplished under general anesthetic and held in plaster fixation. Swelling of the foot is frequently marked and should be combatted by elevation.

Particular care should be taken to regain the curve of the metatarsals. Lateral displacement will not cause permanent difficulty, but plantar angulation or a bony prominence on the weight-bearing surface will cause later difficulty in walking.

Fractures at the Base of the Fifth Metatarsal.—These fractures occur usually when the foot is sharply inverted with the body weight forward on the front part of the foot, as in running. A sudden strain is placed on the peroneus brevis muscle at its insertion in the base of the fifth metatarsal. These injuries are frequently overlooked and diagnosed as sprains. They are characterized by tenderness directly over the base of the fifth metatarsal which is prominent and easily palpated. The treatment consists either of a plaster boot or of an adhesive plaster strapping with a felt doughnut over the fracture site. If the strapping is adequate to prevent a pull on the peroneus brevis the patient is usually able to walk in more or less comfort by the end of the second week. A rigid-soled shoe will make weight-bearing more comfortable and do away with the necessity of plaster fixation.

Occasionally these fractures do not heal by bony union, but in most instances the fibrous union is adequate for function.

"March" Fractures of the Metatarsals.—Crack fractures through the shafts of the second, third or fourth metatarsals may occur during prolonged walking or marching without specific trauma. They are characterized by pain and mild swelling and are frequently unrecognized until a mass of callus appears on the x-ray films. A walking plaster boot for from three to four weeks should be applied when the diagnosis is made early. Late cases may be treated by non-weight-bearing active exercises until the pain and tenderness subside.

FRACTURES OF THE PHALANGES

These are frequently crushing injuries caused by a weight falling on the foot; stubbing the toes against furniture in the dark is another method of injury. The fractures may be accompanied by considerable swelling of the soft parts. If the breaks are in the shafts of the four small toes, adhesive strapping around the affected toe and the one next to it act as a splint may be all that is necessary. If more than one toe is injured a plaster sole for immobilization for a few days is satisfactory. Occasionally a reduction is necessary if the deformity is such that it will interfere in weight-bearing. Restoration of full mobility of the joint is not of great importance. Three or four weeks is usually all that is necessary for protection but tenderness may persist for some time thereafter.

DISLOCATIONS AT THE METATARSO-TARSAL JOINTS

Rarely cases are seen where the entire row of metatarsals is displaced on the tarsus. The deformity is marked. In early dislocations reduction under an anesthetic is relatively simple. Immobilization with no weight-bearing for two or three weeks should be all that is necessary. Dislocations of the toes are not common but occasionally occur and are usually easily reduced.

References

American College of Surgeons: *An Outline of the Treatment of Fractures,* 5th Ed., 1954.

BANCROFT and MARBLE: *Surgical Treatment of the Motor Skeletal System,* 2nd Ed., Philadelphia, J. B. Lippincott Co., 1951.

BLOUNT, WALTER B.: *Fractures in Children,* Baltimore, The Williams & Wilkins Co., 1954.

KEY and CONWELL: *Fractures, Dislocations and Sprains,* 5th Ed., St. Louis, The C. V. Mosby Co., 1951.

MAGNUSON and STACK: *Fractures,* 5th Ed., Philadelphia, J. B. Lippincott Co., 1949.

SMITH, F.M.: *Surgery of the Elbow,* Springfield, Charles C Thomas, 1954.

WATSON-JONES: *Fractures and Joint Injuries,* 3rd Ed., Baltimore, The Williams & Wilkins Co., 1944.

Index

A

ABDOMINAL distention, 149
  signs, 149
Abnormal mobility 26–28
Acetabular fragment, 172
  rim, 170
Acetabulum, 171–172
  fractures of, 156
Achilles tendon, 205
Acromial fractures, 68
  fragments, 65
Acromioclavicular joint, dislocations of, 62, 68–72
Acromion, 65, 66, 68, 69, 96
Adductor canal, 56
  muscle, 173
Adhesions, 23
Adhesive plaster for sole, 57
  for strapping, 46–48, 138, 185
    of ankle, 46
    of chest, 47, 147
    of knee, 47
    of wrist, 48
  for traction, 55
Aeroplane splint, 79, 82
Age of patient, 10, 23, 31, 157
Alignment, changes in, 25
American College of Surgeons, Fracture Committee of, 30
Anatomical neck of humerus, fractures of, 74–75, 89
  snuff-box, 133
Anatomy, normal, of ankle, 197–198
  of elbow, 94–96
  of hip, 156–160
  of shoulder, 60
  of wrist, 124–125
Anesthesia, danger of, 31
  general, 32, 39
  local, 32, 54

(210)

Angulation, 13, 62, 166, 168
Angle, aspiration of, 54
  dislocations of, 200
  fractures of, 194–202
  strapping of, 46–47
Ankylosis, danger of, 138
Antecubital fossa, 99, 109, 113
Antitoxin, tetanus, 39, 60
Aponeurosis of triceps, 112
  of quadriceps, 183
Aponeurotic expansion of quadriceps, 182
Apparatus, construction of, 35
  for traction suspension, 55–57
  Roger Anderson, Haynes, Stader, 175, 192
Application of splints, 42–45
Arm, lengthening of, 88
  shortening of, 76, 89, 96, 102
  splint for, 45
  uninjured, confinement of, 101
Arterial spasm, 98
Artery, brachial, 77, 96
Arthritis, traumatic, 156, 202, 204, 205, 207
Aseptic necrosis, 163, 171, 203
Aspiration of ankle, 54
  of elbow, 52
  of joints, 52–54, 109, 110, 184, 187
Australian traction, 35, 175. See also Russell.
Avulsion of extensor tendon, 143
Axillary nerve, 84, 88.
  pad, 92
  vessels, 77
Axis, 12
  changes in, 25, 27, 185

B

BACK, exercises for, 150
Backache, 148, 151

Index

Bandages, 43
  constricting, 22, 97, 98, 99
  elastic, 56, 192
  figure-of-eight, 63
  for traction, 42–45
  plaster-of-Paris, 45, 48
  pressure, 206
  Velpeau, 64
Baseball fingers, 143
Baths, whirlpool, 40
Bed, Gatch, 149
  rest in, 36, 152, 154
  sores, 151
Bennett fractures, 138
Biceps, 76
  displacement of long head of, 90
Bicipital fascia, 96
  groove, 90
Binder, flannel, 47
Bladder, damage, 154, 155
  infection, 151
Blood clotting, 20
  extravasation of, 15, 19, 20, 21, 25
  in joint, 21, 109
  infiltration in tissues, 67, 109
  vessels, axillary, 77
    injuries to, 10, 16, 19, 21, 31. *See also* Specific injuries.
    popliteal, 182
    subclavian, 62, 77
    synovial, 160
    thrombosis of, 21
Bone, bleeding of, 19
  bowing of, 121
  cancellous, 22, 126, 187
  chips, 192
  cortical, 22
  decalcified, 37
  formation in muscle, 101
  graft, 134, 192
  overgrowth or overproduction of, 109, 110, 113, 115
  repair of, 19–22
  sesamoid, 183
  type of, 22
Bone-forming period, 109

Bony irregularity, 16, 25
Brace of ankle, 195
  caliper, 168
  spinal (Taylor), 150
Brachial artery, 77, 96
  plexus, 63, 77, 84, 85
  vein, 77
Brachialis anticus, fibers of, 114
  fibers, 25, 101, 113
  tearing of, 113
Bryant's triangle, 159, 166
  suspension, 173, 177

C

CALCANEOUS, 200, 202
  fractures of, 205–207
Calcification in ligaments, 115
  absorption of, 20
Calcium, absorption of, 20
  available, 21
  concentration of, 20
  deposition of, 20
Caliper brace, 168, 176
Callus, 20, 21, 23, 28, 37, 166, 168, 208
Canal, adductor (Hunter's), 56
  carpal, 136
    removal of bone from, 137
Cancellous bone, 22, 126, 187
Capitate, 135, 136
Capitellar epiphysis, 104
Capitellum, 94, 104, 116
Cardiac disease, 31
Carpal bones, dislocations of, 135–137
  fractures of, 21, 135
  canal, 136
    removal of bone from, 137
  ligament, 136
  scaphoid, fractures of, 21, 132–135
    removal of, 134
Carpo-radial joint, 136
Carpus, fractures of, 132–135
Carrying angle, 96
Cartilage, epiphyseal, of elbow, 107

Index

Cartilage, epiphyseal, of knee, 182
  of wrist, 131
  semilunar, 187
Casings, plaster-of-Paris, 48–52
Cell, osteogenetic, 20
  red blood, 155
  white blood, 19
Cervical vertebrae, dislocations of, 152–153
Chest injuries, 147
  strapping of, 47, 147
Childbirth, interference with, 156
Children examination of, 15
  injuries common in, 61, 79, 94, 104, 105, 110, 114, 118, 120, 122, 173, 181, 189
  symptoms of, 23
Chip, avulsed, 13
  fractures, 143
  grafts, 192
Circulation, 16, 20, 21, 22, 32, 41, 52
Circulatory damage, 33–34, 175. *See also* Specific injuries.
Clavicle, dislocations of, 69–72
  fractures of, 61–65
  subperiosteal excision of, 71
Cleansing of wound, 37–38
Clinical observations, importance of, 18
Closed reduction, 32, 33. *See also* Specific injuries.
Closure of wound, delayed, 38
Clotting of blood, 20
Collar, leather, 153
  plaster, 153
  Shantz, 153
College of Surgeons, American, 30
Colles' fractures 11, 124–130
  reverse, 130
Color, 16
  of fingers, 98, 99
Comminuted fractures, 12, 19, 36, 166, 173, 176, 201, 205
Commoli's sign, 66
Compensation cases, 18
  laws, 13

Complications of carpus fractures, 137
  of hip fractures, 162, 163, 164
  of lower end of radius, 127, 132
  of metacarpals, 138
  of ribs, 147
  of shoulder dislocations, 89–90
  of supracondylar fractures, 101
Compound fractures, 12, 31, 37–39
Compression fractures, 148, 149, 150, 205
Condyle, humeral, external or lateral, 104–105, 118
  internal or medial, 105
  tibial, external or lateral, 185
  internal or medial, 185
Condyles, 102, 185, 187
Confidence of patient, 11, 15
Constricting bandages, 22, 97, 98, 99
Cooperation of patient, 10, 11, 14, 31
Coracoclavicular ligaments (conoid, trapezoid), 62, 65, 68, 69, 72
Coracoid, 65, 67, 68, 69, 71, 83, 88
  fractures, 68
Cord, spinal, 148
  injury to, 148, 150, 153
Coronoid process, 113
  fractures of, 113–114
Cortical bone, 20, 22
Costoclavicular ligament (rhomboid), 62
Count, white cell, 19
Countertraction, 30, 85, 128, 152
Coxa vara deformity, 166
  displacement of fragments, 159
Crepitus, 16, 25, 27, 66, 189
Crucial ligaments, 188
Cuirass, plaster, 152

D

DEATH, instant, 153
  tissue, 19, 20, 21

Index

Debridement, 38
Decalcified bone, 37
Deformed joint, 110
Deformity, 10–12, 171, 189. See also Specific injuries.
  angular, 79, 117, 138, 164
  coxa vara, 166
  definition and cause of, 25
  "gunstock," 101
  increase of, 64, 187
  in relation to diagnosis, 14–15, 16, 27
    function, 73, 139, 141
  old, 14
  persistent, 68, 132
  prevention of, 102, 104
  recurrence of, 120, 126
  residual, 28, 123, 130, 179, 188
  "silver fork," 125, 131
  types of, 25
  varus, 157
Delayed union, 91, 122, 123, 164, 175, 190
Deltoid, 65, 76, 77, 84, 88, 91
  curve, 83
  weakness of, 84
Deposition of calcium, 20
Diagnosis, 13–18. See also Specific injuries.
Discoloration, at elbow, 108
  of skin, 25
Disease(s), cardiac, 31
  respiratory, 31
  systemic, 22
Disinfectants, 38
Dislocations, 25, 27
  acromioclavicular, 62, 68–72
  ankle, 200
  carpal bones, 135–137
  clavicle, 68–72
  elbow, 17, 105, 114, 119
  forearm bones, 105
  hip, 170–171
  lunate, 132, 135–137
  metatarsotarsal joint, 209
  recurrence of, 84, 88
  shoulder, 83–88
  vertebra, 152–153
Displacements, 13–19, 24, 25
  kinds of, 13. See also Specific injuries.
Distention, abdominal, 149
Dorsolumbar junction, 145
Drainage, circulatory, 99
  lymphatic, 96
  venous, 96–97
Dressings, plaster-of-Paris, 48, 73
  removable, 48
Drill, hand or motor, 56
Drilling, multiple, 192
Duga's sign, 84

E

Ecchymosis, 15, 25, 164. See also Specific injuries.
Economic handicap, 12
Edema, 21, 32, 96, 201
Edematous infiltration, 25
  swelling, 27
Elastic bandage, 56
Elbow joint, aspiration of, 52
  discoloration at, 108
  dislocations of, 17, 105, 114–119
  fractures at, 94–102
  stiff, 102
"Electric treatments," 11
Emergency splints, 42–45
  treatment, 29–31, 38. See also First aid.
Endocrine disturbances, 22
Epicondyle, internal, 115
  fractures of, 105–107
  lateral, 54
Epicondyles, 94, 96, 102, 114
Epiphyseal cartilage of elbow, 107
  of knee, 182
  of wrist, 131
  ossification of, 21
  line of femur, 175, 181
Epiphysis, 21, 182
  separation of, capitellar, 104
    lower femoral, 171–182
      humeral, 105, 107–108
      radial, 130–132

Index

Epiphysis, separation of, internal condyle, 115
  of tibia or fibula, 201
  upper femoral, 168–170
    humeral, 79–81
    radial, 110
Equipment, 32, 37
Esophagus, 73
Examination of patient, 14, 17, 31, 34
  by x-ray, 17, 39
  example of, 17
  general, 14
  local, 14
  rough, 22
Exercises, 75, 103, 150, 180
  for back, 150
  pendulum, 78
Extensor longus pollicis, 54
  muscles, 104, 120
  tendon, 143
Extravasation of blood, 15, 19, 20, 21, 25
Extremity, lower, injuries to, 157–209
  upper, injuries, to, 61–145
  usefulness of, 10
Exudate, inflammatory, accumulation of, 19

F

FACTORS influencing healing, 20–22
Fascia, 19, 25, 31, 120
  bicipital, 96
  of elbow and forearm, slitting of, 100
Felt yokes, Magnuson, 102–103
Femoral epiphysis, lower, separation of, 179–180
  upper, separation of, 169–170
  head, 156, 170, 171
Femur, 21, 29, 35, 56
  fractures of head, 156
    of lower extremity, 178–180
    of neck, 21, 159, 163
    of shaft, 172–177
    of upper extremity, 157–172

Fibers, brachialis, 25, 101, 113
  anticus, 114
Fibroblasts, 20
Fibrocartilage, 73
Fibrosis, 21, 67, 78
Fibrous tissue, 23, 100. *See also* Specific injuries.
  union, 106, 112, 192, 195, 196, 208
Fibula, 54
  fractures of shaft of, 189–193, 199
Fibular neck, 187
Figure-of-eight dressings, 99
Finger joint, stiff, 12
Fingers, anesthesia of, 136
  baseball, 143
  color of, 98, 99
  fracture of, 12, 138–145
  function of, 121
  motion of, 12, 33, 98, 128, 135–136, 142
  sensation in, 98
  temperature of, 98, 99
  use of, 137
First aid treatment (spinal injuries), 148. *See also* Emergency.
Fixation, 37
  internal 38. *See also* Internal splints.
Flannel binder, 47
Flat foot, traumatic, 199, 201
Flexor brevis, 144
  muscle, 105, 120
  tendon, 136, 143, 144
Fluid in joint, 52, 109
Fluids, intravenous, 39
  tissue, 20
Follow-up, importance of, 41
Foot, injuries to, 203–209
Foot-drop, prevention of, 57
Forearm, 36
  bones, dislocation of, 105
  injuries to, 120–123
Fracture Committee of American College of Surgeons, 30
Fractures, classification of, 12–13

Index

Fractures, comminuted, 13, 19, 36, 166, 173, 176, 201, 205
  compound, 12, 31, 37–39
  compression, 148, 149, 150, 205
  definition of, 9–12
  diagnosis of, 13–18
  confirmation by x-ray, 17
  fracture-dislocations, 138
  "greenstick," 19, 25, 120, 121
  impacted, 157, 159, 160, 163
  line, 160, 189
  oblique, 13, 33, 36, 65, 140, 141, 143, 173, 189, 194, 195
  repair of bone in, 19–22
  simple, 12, 31
  spiral, 13, 29, 140, 189, 191, 194
  stellate, 65, 111, 182
  symptoms and signs of, 24–28
  transverse, 13, 65, 140, 141, 173, 174, 189, 190
  trauma associated with, 10–11, 19
  unsplinted, effect of, 31
Fragments, 13, 21, 24. *See also* Specific injuries.
  acetabular, 172
  apposition of, 163
  displacement of, 21, 159, 173
  fixation of, 37
  impacted, 13, 157
  multiple, 21
  shift of, 13, 24
Frame, 149
Frames for traction, 55–57
"Frog" position, 174
Frölich syndrome, 169
Function, impairment of, 24, 27. *See also* Specific injuries.
  maintenance of, during treatment, 33
  restoration of, 32
Functional result, 11
Functions, dissimilar, 11
  motor investigation of, 16
  sensory investigation of, 16

G

GASTROCNEMIUS muscle, 178, 182, 198, 200
Gatch bed, reversed, 149
Gauntlet, plaster, 51, 128, 133, 134, 138
Girdle pains, 149
Glenoid, 65, 66, 68, 84
  fracture of, 89
  ligament, 144, 145
Golf, 41
Graft, 134, 192
Granulation tissue, 20, 21, 28, 32
Greater tuberosity, 76
  fractures of, 81–83, 89
"Greenstick" fracture, 19, 25, 120, 121
Grip, interference with, 141
Growth, disturbance, 101, 108, 132, 170, 182, 201
  interference with, 21
"Gunstock" deformity, 101

H

HAND injuries to, 138–145
  use of, 128
Handicap, economic, 12
Haynes apparatus, 175
Head halter, traction by, 152, 153
Healing powers, poor, 21
  processes, 20–22
Heat, 39, 40. *See also* Specific injuries.
Heel, 43
"Heel-in-the-axilla," 85
Hemarthrosis, 25, 52, 108–109, 113, 133, 185
Hematocrit, 173
Hematoma, 127
  organizing, 25, 28, 54
  retroperitoneal, 149
  subungual, 143
Hemorrhage, 13, 20, 21, 66, 77, 82, 96, 120, 173, 189
  control of, 59
Hemothorax, 147

Index

Hip joint, dislocations of, 170–171
    fractures at, 157–172
History, 31, 126
    example of, 16
    importance of, 13, 14, 16
Hot soaks, 129, 142, 201
Humeral axis, 114
    head, 66, 84
Humerus, 35, 114, 118
    anatomical neck of, fractures of, 74–75, 89
    lower extremity of, fractures of, 94–108
    shaft of, fractures of, 91–93
    upper extremity of, dislocations of, 83–89
        fractures of, 74–83
Hunter's canal, 56
Hypesthesia, 84

I

Iliac ala, 154
    crests, 154
Iliopsoas, 173
Ilium, fractures of, 154
Immobilization, 32, 33, 51
    improvised means of, 45
    of fracture into joint, 23
    temporary, 45
Impacted fractures, 79, 160, 162
    fragments, 13, 157
Impaction, 75, 78, 124, 127, 157, 161
Impairment of function, 24, 27
Individual, characteristics of, 14
    condition of, 14
    importance of, 10
Infection, 21, 34, 37, 38
    bladder, 151
Inflammation, local, 19
Infraspinatus, 82
Injection of novocaine, 54, 127, 147
    technique for, 54
Injury, extent of, 19, 20
    site of, 21

Internal fixation, 37. *See also* Specific injuries.
    organs, injured, 10
    splints, 37
Interphalangeal joints, dislocations of, 145
Interposition of muscle fibers, 22, 29, 63
    of soft parts, 23, 37, 91, 92, 177
Intertrochanteric fractures, 164–166
    line, 160
    region, 21
Intracapsular fractures, 157–164
Intramedullary pins, 142
Intravenous fluids, 39
Ischemic paralysis, 97, 101, 120
Ischial tuberosity, 43, 159
Ischium, fractures of, 154–156

J

Jacket, plaster, 150, 152
Japanese basket-weave splints, 143
Jig-saw work, 40
Joint, acromioclavicular, 57, 62, 68–72
    ankle, 54
    capsule, 25, 52, 73, 83, 84, 108, 109, 145, 171, 184, 185
        aspiration of, 52–54, 109, 110, 187
        cavity of, 52
        distended, 108
        tearing of, 109, 113, 114
    carporadial, opening of, 136
    deformed, 110
    elbow, 52, 94–119
    fluid in, 109
    fracture into, 21, 138, 187
    hip, 157–172
    interphalangeal, 145
    knee, 47, 178–188
    metacarpocarpal, 138
    metacarpophalangeal, 144–145
    metatarsophalangeal, 51

Index

Joint, metatarsotarsal
  midtarsal, 197
  radio-ulnar, 126, 130
  sacro-iliac, 156
  shoulder, 57, 74–90
  sternoclavicular, 72–73
  stiff, 40, 102, 104, 138
  subtalar, 197, 205, 206
  wrist, 36, 48, 51, 54, 124–137

K

Kirschner wire, 69, 99, 103, 122, 128, 130
Knee, aspiration of, 54
  injuries at, 178–188
  strapping of, 47
Knitting, 40
Knots for traction bandages, 42–43, 57
Knuckle, dropped, 141
Kocher maneuvers, 86
Kyphosis, 149

L

Labium, 43
Lacerations, 60
Lacertus fibrosus, 96
Laminectomy, 151
Laws, compensation, 13
Leadbetter method, 161
  sign, 161
Leather collar, 153
Leg, casings, 51
  fractures of, 30, 36, 157–207
  shortening of, 27
  splinting of, 43–44
Length, 12
  changes in, 25
  maintenance of, 31
Lengthening of arm, 88
Lesser tuberosity, fractures of, 83
Ligament(s), calcification in, 115
  carpal, 136
  conoid, 62
  coracoclavicular, 62, 65, 68, 69, 72
  costoclavicular (rhomboid), 62

Ligaments(s), crucial, 188
  crucial, 188
  elbow, 115
  glenoid, 144–145
  inferior tibiofibular, 197, 199, 201, 202
  medial collateral (knee), 185, 187
  orbicular, 116, 118
  radial collateral, 133
  radiolunate, 135
  sternoclavicular, 73
  tibiofibular, 199
  torn, 133, 185
  trapezoid, 62
  vertebral, anterior, 149
Ligamentum teres, 160, 171
Local inflammation, 19
Lower extremity, injuries to, 157–209
  femoral epiphysis, separation of, 181–182
Lumbar curve, loss of, 149
  vertebrae, 149
Lunate, dislocation of, 132, 135–137
Lymph, circulation of, 22
Lymphatic circulation, 20
  drainage, 96

M

Magnuson felt yokes, 102–103
Malleoli, 197
  fractures of, 194–201
Malleolus, lateral, fractures of, 194
  medial, 157
  fractures of, 195–197
"March" fractures of metatarsals, 208
Massage, 40. *See also* Specific injuries.
Median nerve, 77, 114, 127, 136
Medicolegal cases, 14, 18
Metacarpal, first, fracture of, 138–140
  head, 145
  angulation, 140

Metacarpals, 138–142
 dislocations of, 144–145
 fractures of, 140–142
 shortening of, 140
Metacarpocarpal joint, fracture-dislocations, 138
Metacarpophalangeal joint, dislocations of, 144–145
Metatarsals, fractures of, 207–208
 "March" fractures, 208
Metatarsophalangeal joints, 51
Metatarsotarsal joints, dislocations at, 209
Mid-palmar crease, 51, 128, 134
Midtarsal joint, 197
Missiles, fractures caused by, 21
Mobility, 11
 abnormal, 26, 28
Morphine, 39
Motion, arc of, 25. *See also* Specific injuries.
 at fracture site, 22, 24
 false point of, 16–25, 27, 166, 189
 forced, passive, 101
 in fingers, 33
 lack of, 14
 limitation of, 25, 27
 limited, 12
 loss of, 27
 range of, 11, 25, 27
 voluntary, 40
Multangular (trapezium), 138
Multiple drilling, 192
 fracture lines, 201
Muscle(s) action, voluntary, 40
 adductor, 173
 biceps, 76, 90
 bruised, 10, 152
 extensor, 104, 120
 fibers, interposition of, 22, 29, 63
  replacement by fibrous tissue, 101
 formation of bone in, 101
 gastrocnemius, 178, 182, 198, 200, 205

Muscle(s) action, injury of, 19, 21, 30, 31, 63
 peroneus brevis, 208
 pull, 31, 33, 105
 quadriceps, 185
 spasm, protective, 20, 24, 31, 32, 149
 tearing of, 152
 thigh, 173
 triceps, 91, 112, 114, 116
 vastus intermedius, 173
Myositis ossificans, 101, 114

N

NAIL (finger), drilling of, 143
 traction through, 143
 intramedullary, 176
 Smith-Petersen, 162, 164, 170
Nails, 103. *See also* Pins.
Navicular of carpus, fractures of, 132–135
Neck, injuries of, 152, 153
 of radius, fractures of, 110–111
Necrosis, aseptic, 163, 171, 203
Nélaton's line, 159, 166
Neoplasm, 25
Nerve(s), axillary, 84, 88
 injuries, 10, 14, 16, 19, 31
  anesthesia from, 84
 intercostal, 147
 median, 77, 114, 127, 136
 musculospiral, 91
 peripheral, 16, 36
 peroneal, 187
 popliteal, 182
 radial, 91, 92, 93, 109, 114
 root signs, 149
 sciatic, 171
 supraclavicular, 63
 ulnar, 56, 77, 104, 106, 112
90–90–90 position, 167
Nonunion, 23, 91, 92, 93, 122, 123, 133, 134, 160, 161, 163, 164, 175, 190
Novocaine, injection of, 54, 127, 147
 technique for, 54

Index

O

OBLIQUE fractures, 13, 33, 36, 65, 140, 141, 143, 173, 189, 194, 195
Occupation of patient, 10, 11
Occupational therapy, 41
Odontoid process, 153
Olecranon, 37, 54, 56, 71, 78, 92, 94, 96, 99, 102, 104, 111, 114, 116
  fossa, 114
  fractures of, 111–113
Open reduction, 36–37. See also Specific injuries.
  delayed, 37
  replacement, epiphysis, 132
Operative procedures, 36–39. See also Specific injuries.
Orbicular ligament, 116, 118
Osseous tissue, 101
Ossification of epiphyseal cartilage, 21
  premature, 21
Osteogenetic cell, 20
Osteomyelitis, 37
Overgrowth of bone, 109–110, 113, 115
Overpull, 13, 92
Overriding, 13, 29, 31. See also Specific injuries.

P

PAIN, 14, 24, 25, 27, 31, 52, 55. See also Specific injuries.
Pains, girdle, 149
Palpation, 15, 25, 27
Paralysis, 151, 152
  ischemic, 97, 101, 120
  Volkmann's, 97, 99, 101, 120, 190
Paravertebral block, 147
Patella, 37, 183, 184, 197
  fractures of, 182–185
Pathology. See Specific injuries.
Patient, age of, 10, 22, 31
  confidence of, 15
Patient, cooperation of, 10, 11, 14, 31
  evaluation of, 31
  examination of, 14, 17
  general condition of, 14, 31
  history of, 13, 14, 16
  temperament of, 10, 11, 14
Pectoralis major, 76
Pegs, 103, 196
Pelvic girdle, injuries to, 154–156
Pelvis, shape of, 156
Pendulum exercises, 78
Penicillin, administration of, 38
Periarticular swelling, 143
Periosteal attachment, 82
Periosteum, 10, 19, 21, 23, 195
Peripheral nerves, 16
Peroneal nerve, 187
Peroneus brevis muscle, 208
Phalanges of foot, dislocations of, 209
  fractures of, 208
  of hand, dislocations of, 145
  fractures of, 142–144
Phalanx of finger, 12
  of toe, 12
  proximal, of thumb, 134, 139, 140
Physical therapy, 40. See also Specific injuries.
Pin, insertion of, 175
Pins, 34, 36, 37, 142, 162. See also Nails.
  Steinman, 164, 172
Place of accident, importance of, 13
Plaster, adhesive. See Adhesive.
Plaster-of-Paris bandages, 45, 48
  boots, 51, 192, 195, 199, 201, 202, 203, 206, 208
  casings, 36, 48–52
  circular, 51, 99, 121, 128, 185, 190
  collar, 153
  cuirass, 152
  cutting instruments, 52
  gauntlet, 51, 128, 133, 134, 138

Plaster-of-Paris bandages, "hanging," 92
  jacket, 150, 152
  removal of, 52
  spicas, 79, 156, 161, 162, 163, 164, 174, 175, 178
  splints, 48–52, 81, 120, 141
Plate, 142, 176
Platysma, 63
Plexus, brachial, 63, 84, 85
Pneumothorax, 147
Popliteal nerves, 182
  vessels, 182
Pott's fracture, 199–201
Prognosis. See Specific injuries.
Pronator radii teres, 120, 122
Protective spasm, 20, 24, 31, 32, 149
Pubis, fractures of, 154–156
Pulse, radial, 98, 99, 100
Pulses, 16

Q

QUADRICEPS, 185
  aponeurosis of, 183
  aponeurotic expansion of, 182
  tendon, 183

R

RADIAL head, 54
  dislocation of, 116–118, 123
  fracture of, 17, 25, 27, 108–110, 115
  fragments of, 106
  subluxation of, 118
  pulse, 98, 99, 100
  styloid, 125, 126
Radiolunate ligament, 135
Radio-ulnar joint, 127, 130
Radius, 135, 136
  dislocation of, 116
  fractures of, 120–123
    lower extremity of, 124–132
    neck of, 110–111
    upper extremity of, 108–111
Ramus of ischium, 154

Recurrence of deformity, 121, 126
Recurrent dislocations of shoulder, 84, 88
Red blood cells, 155
Reduction, 30, 32, 33. See also Specific injuries.
Reduction, anesthesia for, 54
  closed, 32, 33
  open, 36–37
  time of, 32, 34
Refractures, 121
Rehabilitation, 39–41
Removal of plaster dressings, 52
Repair of bone, factors influencing, 20–22
Replacement of muscle fibers, 101
Respiratory disease, 31
Retroperitoneal hematoma, 149
Reverse Colles' Fracture, 130
Ribs, fractures of, 147
Roger Anderson apparatus, 175
Rotation, changes in, 25. See also Specific injuries.
Russell traction, 35, 36, 92, 164, 167, 175. See also Australian.

S

SAYRE dressing, 64
Scaphoid, 132, 135
Scapula, fracture of, 65–68
Scapular glenoid, 65, 66, 68
  neck, 65, 66, 68
  spine, 65
Sciatic nerve, 171
Screws, 37, 103, 112, 142, 163, 176, 188, 196
Scrotum, 43
Secondary trauma, 19, 22, 29
Semilunar bone, 132
  cartilages, 187
Sesamoid bone, 183
Shantz, collar, 153
Shock, 14, 31, 59, 173
  blocks, 57
  mental, 10, 31
  tissue, 20, 24

Index

Shoulder, 45, 121
  girdle, dislocations of, 68–72
    fractures of, 61–68
  joint, capsule of, 84
    dislocations of, 83–88
    fractures of, 74–90
Sigmoid cavity (lesser), 117
"Silver fork" deformity, 125, 131
Skeletal traction, 34, 56, 93, 139, 142, 152, 167, 178
Skeleton, condition of, 22
Skin, care of, 162
  discoloration of, 25
  injury of, 10, 19, 21
  traction, 34, 55–56, 78, 86, 93, 171
Smith-Petersen nail, 162, 164, 170
Snuff-box, anatomical, 133
Soft part(s), attachments, 21
  damage to, 10, 14, 16, 19, 22, 25, 29, 152, 166
  interposition of, 37, 91, 177
  stretching of, 114. *See also* Specific fractures.
Sores, bed, 151
  pressure, 162
Spasm, arterial, 98
  protective, 20, 24, 31, 32, 149
Spica, plaster, 79, 156, 161, 162, 163, 164, 174, 175, 178
Spinal brace, Taylor, 150
  cord, 152
    damage to, 148, 150, 151, 152, 153
  fusion, 151
Spine, anterior-superior, 156, 159, 197
    inferior-anterior, 154
    superior-anterior, 154
  injuries to, 148–153
  thoracic, 150
  tibial, 188
Spinous process, tenderness over, 148
Splint(s), 32, 33
  aeroplane, 79, 82
  ambulatory, 75
  arm, 45

Splint(s), banjo, 139
  emergency, 42–45
  internal, 37
  Japanese basket-weave, 143
  leg, 42–44
  length of, 33
  molded, 49–51, 92
  padded board, 45
  plaster-of-Paris, 48–52, 141
  shoulder, 64
  sugar tongs, 81, 92, 121, 123, 128, 130, 190, 194, 198, 200, 201
  T, 64
  techniques, Roger Anderson, Haynes, Stader, 192
  Thomas, 30, 42–45, 175
  Tobruk, 44
Splinting, 24, 39
  immediate, 22
  temporary, 30
Sprains, 107
  foot, 194
  wrist, 133
Stader apparatus, 175
Stave fractures, 138
Steel plates, 37
Steinman pin, 164, 172
Stellate fractures 65, 111, 182
  ganglion blocks, 100
Sternoclavicular joint, dislocation of, 72–73
  ligament, 73
Sternum, 72
Stiff joint, 40, 102, 104, 138
Stockings, Unna paste, 192
Strapping, adhesive, 46–48
  ankle, 46
  chest, 47
  knee, 47
  wrist, 48
Styloid, radial, 125
  ulnar, 124, 125
Subclavian vessels, 62 ,64, 77
Subcoracoid dislocations, 81, 83–88
Subcutaneous tissue, 19
Subdeltoid bursa, 82

Index

Subglenoid dislocations, 88
Subluxation, vertebrae, cervical, 153
Subperiosteal excision, 71
    fracture, 189
Subscapularis, 76, 83, 84
Subtalar joint, 197, 205, 206
Subtrochanteric fractures, 166–169
Supinators, 120
Supraclavicular nerves, 63
Supracondylar fractures, 94–102, 108, 114, 178–180
    region, 175
    ridge, 104
Supraspinatus, 76, 82
Suprasternal notch, 150
Surgeons, American College of, 30
Surgical neck (of humerus), 75, 89
    fracture of, 75–79, 89
    technique, 35, 38, 52, 54
Suspension, 33, 36. *See also* Specific injuries.
    apparatus, 55–57, 187
    Bryant's, 173, 177
Swathe, 45, 75, 78, 81, 85, 88, 188
Swelling, 13, 15, 25, 27, 32, 47, 52, 138. *See also* Specific injuries.
    edematous, 25, 27
Symphysis pubis, 150
Symptoms and signs of fractures, 24–28
Synostosis, 110
Synovial vessels, 160
Synovitis, villous, 25
Systemic diseases, 22

T

T FRACTURES of humerus, 102–104
T splint, 64
Talus, 197, 199
    fractures of, 203–205
Tarsus, fractures of, 203–207
Taylor spinal brace, 150
Technique, aseptic, 56
    for injection of novocaine, 54
    in treatment of fractures, 42–57
    splint, Roger Anderson, Haynes, Stader, 192
    surgical, 35, 38
Temperature of extremity, 16
    of fingers, 98, 99
    rise of, 19
Tenderness, bony, 15, 25
    direct, 25, 27
    indirect, 15, 25, 27, 28
Tendon(s) Achilles, 205
    extensor, 143
    flexor, 136, 143, 144
    quadriceps, 183
Tenosynovitis, 25
Terres major, 76
    minor, 82
Tetanus antitoxin, 39, 60
    toxoid, 60
Therapy, occupational, 41
    physical, 40. *See also* Specific injuries.
Thigh, 154, 171, 175
    muscles, 173
    war wounds of, 175
Thomas splint, 30, 42–45, 175
    wrench, 141
Thoracic cage, compression of, 147
    spine, 150
Thrombosis, 21
Thumb, 133, 138, 139, 145
    proximal phalanx of, 134, 139, 140
Tibia, 178, 188, 201
    "greenstick" fracture of, 25
    lower extremity of, fractures of, 201
    posterior lip of, 197
    shaft of, fractures of, 189–193
    upper extremity, fracture of, 185–188
Tibial spine, fractures, of, 188

Index

Tibial spine, tuberosity, 175
Tibiofibular ligament, inferior, 197, 199, 201, 202
  separation of, 199–201
Time of accident, importance of, 14
Tissue, damaged, 19, 21, 25, 38
  deaths, 19, 20, 21
  fibrous, 100, 152
  fluids, 20
  granulation, 20, 21, 28, 32
  infiltration of, 19
  necrosis of, 21
  osseous, 101
  shock, 20, 24
  subcutaneous, 19
Toe joint, motion in, 12
  phalanx of, 12
Toes, fractures of, 208
Tongs, 34, 152
Trachea, 72
Tracheotomy, emergency, 59
Traction, 24, 30, 31, 33, 36, 39, 42–45, 161. *See also* Specific injuries.
  ambulatory, 36
  apparatus, 55–57
  Australian, 35, 175
  continuous, 33
  Russell, 35, 36, 92, 164, 167, 175
  skeletal, 34, 56, 93, 139, 142, 152, 167
  skin, 34, 55–56, 86, 171
  wire, 92
Transportation, 30, 44
  careless, 22, 29
Transverse fractures, 13, 65, 92, 141, 173, 174, 189
  process, fractures of, 151
Trapezium, 138
Trapezoid (coracoclavicular) ligaments, 62
Trauma, 10, 170, 180
  secondary, 19, 22, 29
Traumatic arthritis, 156, 202, 204, 205, 207
  flat foot, 199, 201

Treatment, 29–41. *See also* Specific fractures.
  choice of, 12, 31
  "electric" 11
  emergency, 29–31, 38
  individual differences in, 10, 11
  methods of, 32
  permanent, 31–39
  principles of, 29–41
Triceps, 91, 112, 114
  aponeurosis of, 112
  aponeurotic expansion of, 112, 116
Trochanter, greater, 156, 159
  lesser, 166, 173
Trochlea, 105, 113
Trunk, injuries to, 147–156
Tuberculosis, 25
Tuberosity of humerus, greater, 76, 81–83, 89
  lesser, 83
  ischial, 43, 159

U

ULNA, 102, 105, 116, 120, 122, 123, 125, 128
  fractures of, 111–114, 116, 120–122, 123
Ulnar head, dislocation of, 122
  nerve, 56, 77, 104, 106, 112
  shaft, angulation, 116
  styloid, 124, 125
Union, 91, 93
  bony, 112, 138, 163, 164
  delayed, 23, 91, 93, 164, 175, 190
  failure of, 75, 91, 113, 133
  fibrous, 106, 112, 192
Unna paste stockings, 192
Upper extremity, injuries to, 61–145
  femoral epiphysis, separation of, 179–180
Urethral damage, 154, 155
Urine, 155

V

Valgus position, 157, 159, 163
Varus deformity, 157, 165
Vastus intermedius, 173
Velpeau bandage, 64
Venous drainage, 96–97
Vertebra, 148, 149, 151, 152
  cervical, 152, 153
    dislocations of, 152–153
  lumbar, 149
  subluxation of, 153
Vertebral body, fractures of, 148–151, 205
  ligament, anterior, 149
Vitallium nail (Smith-Petersen), 162, 164, 170
Volkmann's paralysis, 97, 99, 101, 120, 190

W

Weaving, 40
Whirlpool baths, 40
White cell count, 19
Whitman method, 172
Wires (for reduction and traction), 34, 35–36, 69, 78, 92, 104, 112, 152, 178, 188. *See also* Specific fractures.
Wires, insertion of, 56
  intramedullary, 64, 112, 142, 176
  Kirschner, 69, 103, 121, 122, 128, 130
  removal of, 57
Wood-carving, **40**
Wound, delayed closure of, 38
Wrench, Thomas, 141
Wrist, 36, 45, 51, 54
  injuries at, 124–137
  sprain of, 133
  strapping of, 48
Wristlet, 128

X

X-ray pictures, 11 17–18, 25, 29, 30, 31, 39, 41. *See also* Specific fractures.

Y

Y fractures of humerus, 102–104
Yokes, Magnuson felt, 102–103

NO LONGER THE PROPERTY
OF THE
UNIVERSITY OF R.I. LIBRARY

SF56
617.15